D1577081

Fields of
Courage

Also by Max Davidson

NON-FICTION

It's Not the Winning That Counts
Sorry! The Hardest Word and How to Use It

FICTION

The Wolf
Beef Wellington Blue
Hugger Mugger
Suddenly in Rome
The Greek Interpreter
Well Done, Beef Wellington

Fields of Courage

The Bravest Chapters in Sport

MAX DAVIDSON

Little, Brown

LITTLE, BROWN

First published in Great Britain in 2011 by Little, Brown

Copyright © Max Davidson 2011

The moral right of the author has been asserted.

A CIP catalogue record for this book
is available from the British Library.

ISBN 978-1-4087-0216-1

Typeset in Garamond by M Rules
Printed and bound in Great Britain by
Clays Ltd, St Ives plc

Papers used by Little, Brown are natural, renewable and
recyclable products sourced from well-managed forests and certified
in accordance with the rules of the Forest Stewardship Council.

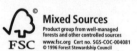

Mixed Sources
Product group from well-managed
forests and other controlled sources
www.fsc.org   Cert no. SGS-COC-004081
© 1996 Forest Stewardship Council
FSC

Little, Brown
An imprint of
Little, Brown Book Group
100 Victoria Embankment
London EC4Y 0DY

An Hachette UK Company
www.hachette.co.uk

www.littlebrown.co.uk

For my late, courageous father, Norman Robson, RIP

And for Hilary – Say Not the Struggle Naught Availeth

Contents

Acknowledgements

My thanks to Little, Brown for publishing a second book on a theme dear to my heart – the inspirational value of sport. I am particularly grateful to my editor Richard Beswick, who shares many of my sporting passions; to Iain Hunt, whose meticulous copy-editing has ironed out many a stylistic gremlin in the manuscript; to Linda Silverman, who has tracked down some great accompanying photographs; to Maddie Mogford, who vetted the text for possible legal complications; and to Rowan Cope, for all her help.

Watching with Mother

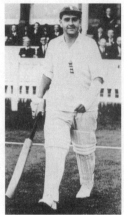

EMPICS

The deprivations of childhood can have long-lasting consequences. I was born in the 1950s, the forgotten decade, the decade of austerity. If I had been born ten years later, into an age of plenty, I would not have had to wait until I was seven years old before my father could afford a television. But then if I had been born ten years later, and grown up with television, I might not be writing this book.

In the Surrey village where I spent the first ten years of my life, the arrival of television – our very own, not just a set in a shop window – had a revolutionary impact. There it was suddenly, in the corner of the sitting-room, when I got home from school, and there, half an hour later, as I sat watching with my mother, was cricket, lovely cricket.

In the weeks and months that followed, I would become addicted to *Crackerjack*, *Hancock's Half Hour*, *Z Cars*, *Hugh and I, Steptoe and Son, I Love Lucy*, all the hit shows of the time. But it was cricket that I got to watch first, and cricket that first wove its magic.

'I think it's the Test match,' said my mother dubiously, fiddling with the aerial. A man with a cricket bat came into focus, then an umpire in a white coat, looking cross. 'Yes, it's the Test match. Imagine that!'

It took at least another six months for me to get my head around the idea of a Test match. 'What are they testing?' I would ask my long-suffering parents. 'When are they going to play the real match?' But on 25 June 1963, there was no time for semantics like that. Fate had decreed that my first taste of Test cricket was one of the most dramatic Tests ever played: England versus West Indies at Lord's, a match for the connoisseurs, a contest of so many twists and turns that a whole book would later be written about it.

I had played cricket in the back garden – where you had to be careful not to hit the ball over the hedge at square leg, which meant asking the fearsome Colonel Goddard for it back – so I knew the rudiments of the game. But, as I could sense from the suppressed excitement in the voice of the commentator, this was 'The Real Thing', played by grown-ups.

I was good at maths, little swot that I was, so the arithmetic of the match was straightforward. England were chasing 234 to win, but running out of wickets – 203 for seven became 219 for eight. Blocking their path to victory, racing in to bowl as if his life depended on it, was the seriously scary Wes Hall. To a boy growing up in a Surrey village in the 1960s, the sight of a black man was an event in itself, on a par with Martians landing in the back garden. But for such a man to launch a cricket ball at a batsman with the velocity of a missile was the stuff of nightmares.

From the moment I set eyes on him, I was in thrall to his terrible beauty. I thought Colonel Goddard was pretty terrifying: he had a voice like a rusty machine-gun and kept bees. Wes Hall began where Colonel Goddard left off. He had something awe-inspiring, elemental, about him.

'What if he killed someone?' I whispered to my mother.

'Don't be silly, dear. It's only a game.'

Only a *game*? Even half a century later, the banality of the answer still has the power to shock. Couldn't she see that what was happening on the TV screen – this demon fast bowler doing his best to batter the English batsmen into submission – had a deeper significance?

With the match scheduled to finish at six o'clock, at ten to six, to my horror, the cricket coverage suddenly stopped and a middle-aged man in a jacket and tie started reading the news.

'But how do we know who won?' I yelped.

'It'll be in the paper tomorrow.'

'Mum, I can't wait for the *paper*.'

Someone at the BBC must have been listening, because the next thing I knew, the telephone on the desk beside the newsreader started ringing. He picked it up, smiled – I can still see that smile to this day – and said: 'Now straight back to Lord's for the conclusion of the Test match.'

I could have hugged him.

And then, like something in a dream, it happened. Another England wicket fell, the West Indies fielders celebrated, everybody looked towards the pavilion, and there, walking down the steps, to a smattering of applause, came a batsman with his arm in plaster.

Crikey! The only other person I had ever seen with his arm in plaster was a boy called Gibson at convent school. He had broken his arm in a playground fall and cried for about six weeks. His gruesome accounts of hospital visits made half the girls in the school cry too. When the cast finally came off, the nuns treated him like a returning war hero.

'That's Colin Cowdrey,' said my mother, with disapproval. 'He shouldn't be batting. Not with a broken arm. He should be resting.'

As a qualified doctor, she knew what she was talking about. But even at the age of seven, eyes glued to the TV screen, I could tell that the situation was not that simple; that doctors don't always know what they are talking about; that there are circumstances when defying medical advice is not foolhardy, but heroic.

With only two balls of the match left, explained the commentator, and Cowdrey as the non-striker, he would probably not have to face Wes Hall – the bowler who had broken his arm earlier in the Test. And so it turned out. The other England batsman, David Allen, blocked the two remaining balls, and the match ended in an honourable draw, with handshakes and smiles all round.

Only a game? Maybe so. But one of such heart-thumping excitement that, in the space of an hour, between homework and baked beans on toast, it had changed my young life, inflaming passions that have never left me.

The first was a passion for Test cricket, that grandest, maddest, subtlest of team sports: a battle of skill and wit stretched out over five whole days. By rights, five-day Test cricket should be a thing of the past, a Victorian relic. Who has five hours to devote to watching men chase a ball about a field, never mind five days? But each time its obituary is pronounced, it rouses itself once more and produces an epic sporting confrontation, like the 2005 Ashes series, which makes all other sports seem trivial.

The second was a particular passion for West Indies cricket. In Wes Hall, gliding in to bowl like a well-oiled machine, I had seen, for the first time in my life, a great athlete. I had seen what it meant to have such a superb physique that you could do things ordinary mortals could not do. But I had also – in Hall and in the West Indies fielders – witnessed something else. Call it spontaneity. Call it exuberance. Call it joy in competition. Whatever it was, I had never seen it in Surrey.

The third, burning just as deeply, was a passion for sporting heroism: the kind of *Boy's Own* courage displayed by Colin Cowdrey, striding down the pavilion steps with his arm in plaster. To the comedy of bat-and-ball, there had been added an element of danger. Only a game? Not with Wes Hall delivering thunderbolts, a nation holding its breath and seven-year-old schoolboys watching mesmerised from the sofa.

Sport in the twenty-first century has fallen prey to the culture of celebrity. New heroes are born every week; put under the microscope; found wanting; discarded. There is a relentless process of trivialisation. But sport, as a force for good, is more durable than its critics allow. For every George Best or Paul Gascoigne – soaring talents that crash and burn as celebrity takes its toll – there is another sporting hero who stays the distance, revered by millions. On the great public stage that their talents have earned for them, they act out parables of endeavour and determination that kindle the imagination.

In my last book, *It's Not the Winning That Counts*, I tried to highlight the role played by chivalry in sport: pinpointing those little acts of good sportsmanship, or gallantry towards an opponent, that embody the Corinthian spirit in which sport ought to be played, but seldom is. This book celebrates another of the great sporting virtues – courage.

The word is sometimes bandied about too easily. Anyone who dies of some painful disease is ritually praised for their courage, as though it were a badge of office. Yet the notion still resonates powerfully, in all walks of life. 'Courage is rightly regarded as the highest of human qualities,' said Winston Churchill, 'because it is the quality that guarantees all the others.' Exactly. And it is one that sportsmen and women have exhibited in particular abundance.

If Colin Cowdrey batting with a broken arm was pretty brave, his heroics seem routine, a mere mention in dispatches, compared with the VC-winning exploits of some of the other sportsmen featured in this book. When the Manchester City goalkeeper Bert Trautmann collected his FA Cup winner's medal in 1956, his head was lolling to one side – X-rays later revealed that he had broken his neck in a goalmouth collision. The pain barriers that some sportsmen have played through are so extraordinary that, as you read about their exploits, you feel physically sick yourself. One New Zealand rugby player insisted on playing on despite a torn scrotum that required twenty-two stitches after the match. The winner of the 1986 Tour de France had shotgun pellets in the lining of his heart, acquired during a hunting accident. Broken ankles, torn cartilages, collapsed lungs: they are all here, like entries in an A & E logbook.

Physically, the heroics of the sports field can seem trivial compared with the heroics of the battlefield or, for that matter, the labour ward. But it is the fact that they are witnessed live by a large audience, in thrall to the drama of the occasion, that explains their iconic power. In the unfolding narrative of a match or a race, a richer human narrative can be glimpsed.

Disabled athletes have demonstrated not just incredible physical resilience, but robustness of spirit, a refusal to be beaten. In the very public arena of sport, their bravery has touched millions, offering a shining example of fortitude in adversity. Their exploits alone could fill a dozen books.

Yet courage resides in the mind as much as the body. The athlete driving his body to extremes of exhaustion to cross the finishing-line first is a magnificent, inspirational spectacle – courage made flesh. But, when the race is run, how do you weigh that kind of courage against the courage to swallow disappointment and put a brave face on defeat?

Some of the bravest figures in sporting history have not been heroic winners, pushing their bodies through the pain barrier, but people who have exhibited courage in other ways – by fighting racism, or by coming out as gay, or by owning up to alcoholism, or to stress-related illnesses. Many were flawed individuals, but it is their strength of character at a time of crisis that we will remember. They were put to the test, in unexpected ways, and responded magnificently.

The same applies to some of the more marginal sporting figures to whom I have paid homage – from the fearless nineteenth-century cricket umpire who waged war on the 'chuckers' to the equally fearless American boxing commentator who quit his sport in disgust in the 1980s.

Some of the women included here were not only brave, but pioneers of their sex, writing their own chapters in social history. When Suzanne Lenglen of France first appeared on court at Wimbledon at 1919, she was doing what no woman had ever previously done at the championships –

showing her calves. Scandalous behaviour! But did it take courage? Without question. One gusty woman was blazing a trail for others. Like Emily Davison, the suffragette who threw herself under the King's horse in the 1913 Derby, Lenglen was using a sporting event to convey a message of larger significance.

Throughout sporting history – and this is why sport, at its best, can command our respect, as well as our affection – men and women have found themselves challenged in ways that transcended the imperatives of winning a race or lifting a trophy. They have had to make moral choices that, because they are public figures, have public consequences. They have not always made the right choices, but when they have taken a stand, their actions have reverberated beyond the narrow confines of sport.

If Muhammad Ali had not been a world-famous sportsman, his refusal to fight in Vietnam would have gone unreported. As it was, he threw down the gauntlet to an entire generation of Americans. His courage at that time cast such a long shadow, was a tipping point of such historical significance, that it is impossible to do it justice in a sporting miscellany of this kind. I have omitted Ali for that reason – just as I have omitted Tommie Smith and John Carlos, whose Black Power salutes at the 1968 Olympics reverberated around the world – for fear of wearying readers with material that is already familiar.

But, even with those omissions, I hope I have been able to demonstrate how sport, for all its faults, has been not only a source of innocent pleasure, but a platform for social change, thanks to the courage of individual sportsmen and women. Who now remembers the name, or even the nationality, of the third man on the podium when Smith and Carlos made their celebrated protest? But he, too, was a moral giant, a man who did his bit for the cause of equality and respect between races.

And I hope I have managed, in these fifty-odd vignettes, to celebrate some of the bravest figures in sporting history: some household names, some long forgotten; but all, without exception, icons of courage.

They dared what others did not dare.

They set an example that still endures.

In short, they inspired.

Bert Trautmann: 'You Should Be Dead'

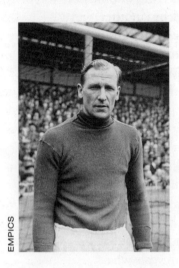

We live in risk-averse times. Wherever we are, whatever we are doing, our health and safety are paramount. Doctors cluck over us. Politicians and civil servants beaver to ensure that we live as long as possible. Life expectancy has never been higher. Compared with our parents, we are in clover. Compared with our grandparents, we are so disgustingly fit and healthy, vaccinated against every disease, insured against every contingency, that we should be dancing in the streets. But there has been – whisper it in the corridors of Whitehall – a price to pay.

It is not a price that can be quantified, or even described with any accuracy. But most of us can sense its existence, there in the background of our cautious, safety-first lives.

And nowhere is it more evident than in sport, that great rococo mirror of society at large.

Watch a Premier League football match on television and you will see the same scenario repeated again and again. A player gets a knock, or pulls a muscle, or develops cramp, and is replaced by another player. The first player limps down the tunnel. The substitute bounds on to the pitch like a rabbit on benzedrine. The commentator waxes lyrical about the millions of pounds of talent that Alex or Rafa or Arsène has on the bench. And the game goes on.

What you hardly ever see, except when a team has used up all its substitutes, is a spectacle that was once commonplace: an injured player having to soldier on because the rules did not allow a replacement. It was not a pretty sight, particularly if the injury was serious, but it stirred the imagination. Football had suddenly become a potent metaphor for life, in which all of us have a role to play, whether we are fit or unfit, and it is our ability to overcome setbacks or handicaps that reveals what we are made of.

In cricket, where substitute fielders are admissible, but not substitute batsmen, you still occasionally see the heirs to Colin Cowdrey emerging from the pavilion, patched up for action. On the South African tour of Australia in 2008–09, the Springbok captain Graeme Smith came out to bat in Sydney with a badly infected elbow and a broken hand, desperate to save the Test for his side. He nearly did it, too, defending doggedly and wincing every time he hit the ball.

It was as if the twenty-first-century SCG, with its state-of-the-art facilities, had suddenly reverted to the Victorian school playing field conjured by Henry Newbolt, in the most famous of cricket poems:

> There's a breathless hush in the Close to-night –
> Ten to make and the match to win –
> A bumping pitch and a blinding light,
> An hour to play, and the last man in.

Cricket, as it so often does, had trained its searchlight on the individual, having to do his bit for his team under the severest pressure. And this individual, hard-as-teak Graeme Smith, was not a man to let a mere broken hand stop him doing his bit for his country.

But football, like rugby, embraced a culture of substitutes long ago. Star players are whisked from the pitch as soon as they feel a tweak in their hamstring, to protect them for the next match. Fresh legs replace tiring legs. Nothing is left to chance in the treatment room.

The England team that won the World Cup in 1966 is imperishable, not least because there were only eleven of them, their names written in the book of their country. Banks, G., Wilson, R., Charlton, J., Moore, R. . . . One for all, all for one. Eleven heroes standing shoulder to shoulder. If England ever win another World Cup, there will be at least fourteen names to have to remember, and they will not be equals. One of them might have played for only five minutes and hardly kicked a ball. The script of the match may have been written by the team physio.

A hero in 2011 is a player who scores a brilliant goal or makes a last-ditch tackle. There is no room left for a different kind of hero. No room for a Bert Trautmann.

Trautmann, born in Bremen, Germany in 1923, and christened Bernhard Carl, was a hero many times over. He was a child of his times. He joined the Hitler Youth and became a champion javelin-thrower. For a time, according to some

accounts, he was an enthusiastic Nazi. By the age of seventeen, he was fighting for his country on the Eastern Front.
He was captured, but escaped, and won the Iron Cross for
bravery. In 1944, now a paratrooper in the Luftwaffe, he
was transferred to the Western Front. Again he was captured, this time by the French Resistance. Again he escaped.
Two American GIs caught him and threatened to execute
him. Trautmann ran away. By the time he was finally captured by the British, and transferred to a POW camp in
Lancashire, he was one of only ninety of his thousand-
strong regiment to survive the war. A hard man, schooled in
hard times.

Embarking on a career as a professional goalkeeper must
have seemed like a holiday in comparison – although not
one without stress.

Trautmann refused an offer of repatriation after the war,
settled in Lancashire and, after a spell at St Helens, signed
for Manchester City in 1949. With the city still scarred by
Luftwaffe bombs, there came a storm of protest. Thousands
demonstrated in the streets. Trautmann received a torrent of
hate mail and shouts of 'Kraut!' and 'Nazi!' from the stands.
But he toughed it out. Others supported him. 'There is no
war in this dressing-room,' declared his club captain Eric
Westwood, a Normandy veteran. A Manchester rabbi wrote
an open letter to a newspaper pleading with people not to
hold one man responsible for the war. And, little by little,
thanks largely to the dignity with which the German conducted himself, the storm blew over. Bernhard became Bert,
with a mangled Lancashire accent. The fans took to him,
not least because he was a superb goalkeeper, the best in the
country.

By the time of the 1956 FA Cup final, against
Birmingham City, Trautmann was at the peak of his career.

He had just won the Football Writers' Association Player of the Year award – the first goalkeeper, and first foreigner, to do so. As a shot-stopper, he was phenomenal, in a class of his own – by the end of his career, he would have saved an incredible 60 per cent of the penalties he faced. He could also throw the ball long distances, turning defence into attack in an instant.

As the day of the final dawned, nobody could have predicted the celebrity that Trautmann was about to achieve, for reasons that had nothing to do with his handling skill.

With his team 3-1 up, and only fifteen minutes remaining, he had to dive at the feet of the oncoming Birmingham City forward Peter Murphy. It was a sickening collision and although Trautmann clutched on to the ball, he was severely concussed and had to be revived by smelling-salts. 'The pain was incredible,' he remembered, years later. 'I couldn't see properly. It was as though I was standing in a thick fog.' Reeling all over the place like a pub drunk, he managed to pull off three stunning saves, but has no memory of them. Manchester City clung on to their 3-1 lead. The Cup was theirs.

When Trautmann staggered up the Wembley steps to collect his winner's medal from the Queen, the extent of his injuries first became apparent. 'Are you all right?' enquired the Duke of Edinburgh. The German's head was at a crooked angle and he was clutching his neck. He felt well enough to attend the post-match banquet, but slept badly and was in severe pain. The next day, he was admitted to St George's Hospital and told it was 'just a crick in the neck'. No medals for the doctor on duty.

The truth emerged only when the goalkeeper got back to Manchester and sought a second opinion. X-rays revealed five damaged vertebrae, one of them cracked in two. Trautmann had broken his neck.

'You should be dead,' the orthopaedic surgeon told him. His convalescence took several months and he missed the start of the following season. He remained a master of his craft, playing for Manchester City until 1964, but a little of the confidence with which he had once dominated the penalty area had gone. 'I can still feel pain in my neck, especially in autumn and winter,' he confided in an interview in 1999. 'Cold and damp seem to affect it.' At the time of writing he lives in retirement in Valencia.

Bert Trautmann has achieved so much, endured so much, that perhaps one should not dwell on a single episode in his life. Just a few months after the 1956 Cup final, his first-born son was killed in a car accident. The war hero and fearless goalkeeper had to face a new test of endurance.

Yet because of the very public nature of sport, and because the FA Cup final is one of the biggest showcases of all, Bert Trautmann will go down in history as the goalie who broke his neck but played on regardless. His courage has become iconic, an inspiration to people who were not even born at the time, a parable of what is possible – in football and in life – if you grit your teeth, stand up and carry on.

Who would have imagined that an ex-Luftwaffe paratrooper could earn such affection in Britain in the years following the Second World War? An act of spectacular physical courage was also a small step on the road to national reconciliation.

In 2004 Trautmann was awarded an honorary OBE for promoting Anglo-German understanding through football.

Later that same year, when the Queen visited Berlin, the veteran German goalkeeper was introduced to her at a concert. 'Ah, Herr Trautmann,' said Her Majesty, normally famous for her lack of interest in football. 'I remember you. Have you still got that pain in the neck?'

Kerri Strug: The Mouse That Roared

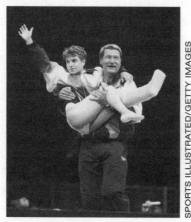

If this book were a waiting room in an A & E department, Bert Trautmann would be at the front of the queue, American gymnast Kerri Strug at the back. A broken neck versus a sprained ankle? No contest. But physical pain is relative: it is how athletes deal with the pain, how they rise to the challenge of the moment, that matters. Parables of sporting courage can take many forms.

Compared with a war-hardened German paratrooper, little Kerri Strug, born in Tucson, Arizona, in 1977, was a character out of a teenage movie, one of those cornball American yarns where no cliché goes unspoken and no heart-string unplucked. She was not only physically diminutive, just four foot nine, but spoke in a squeaky voice that made her sound like a three-year-old blowing up a balloon. Even her surname was oddly unimpressive. It was as if Fate had started to write an epic about Struggle, but ran out of ink.

But Kerri Strug, unquestionably, became a heroine to millions. Ask any American for their all-time favourite Olympic moment and there is a fair chance they will choose this much-loved, much-replayed vignette from the 1996 Olympics in Atlanta. Drama, suspense, comedy, patriotic fervour, athletic brilliance, even a Cold War subtext. It had the lot.

Strug was eighteen at the time of the games, practically a veteran in the precocious world of women's gymnastics. At the Barcelona Olympics four years earlier, she had won a team bronze medal, and been coached by the great Bela Karolyi of Hungary. But when Karolyi retired after the Barcelona games, Strug enjoyed less success with other coaches. She had a bad run of injuries, culminating in a fall from the high bar in 1994, when she landed in a twisted position, had to be stretchered from the gym, then spent long months in rehab. But her luck was slowly changing. She made a full recovery and, in the build-up to Atlanta, got another boost when Karolyi came out of retirement to help her prepare for the games.

In the seven-woman American team, Strug was the quiet one, overshadowed by star performers like Dominique Dawes and Shannon Miller. But as in all team sports, it is often not the stars that make the headlines, but someone from the chorus line, a mouse that roars.

The events of 23 July that catapulted Strug to national stardom were simultaneously perfectly simple and so fiendishly complicated that you needed a pocket calculator to make sense of them. The simple part was the politics. The team gymnastics event at Olympics had long been dominated by the Russians. The Americans had never won it. Now, suddenly, as the event had reached its climax, they had a chance to put one over on their great rival. Everything came down to the final rotation on the final day of competition. The Americans had stormed into an early lead but, after one of their team messed up her vaults, the pressure was suddenly on Strug, the last member of the team to vault.

So far, so simple. Now for the pocket calculator. Strug, who was allowed two vaults, stumbled as she landed at the end of her first one, injured her ankle in the process, and registered only 9.162 on the scoreboard. Was it enough? The NBC commentator had told viewers that Strug needed to score 9.493 or better to make sure of winning gold for the Americans. Bela Karolyi later said he thought the figure was nearer 9.6. In fact, when the final figures were totted up, Strug had already done enough, and there was no need for her to jump again. But how could she be sure of that?

Under the rules of the competition, an interval of only thirty seconds was allowed between vaulting attempts.

'Do we need this?' she asked Karolyi, grimacing in pain.

'Kerri, we need to go one more time,' said the coach. 'We need to go one more time for the gold. You can do it, you better do it.'

So Strug did it. 'This is the Olympics,' she would later tell the media. 'This is what you dream about from when you are five years old. I wasn't going to stop.' Limping as she walked to the end of the runway, she ran thirty yards, vaulted, landed on both feet, then immediately had to transfer her weight on to her one good foot, hopping up and down like a child wanting to go the lavatory. It was inelegant, but it did the trick: it satisfied the requirements of the traditional post-vault pose. The vault scored 9.712

and, whichever pocket calculator you were using, that was good enough to secure gold for the Americans.

As the gymnast collapsed on the mat in tears, holding her damaged ankle, a whole nation went mad.

'In my thirty-five years of coaching, I have never seen such a moment,' Karolyi told the world press afterwards. 'People think these girls are fragile dolls. They're not. They're courageous.'

The thirty thousand crowd in the Georgia Dome cheered the gymnast to the echo. The Russians looked stunned, as if they had been the victims of a confidence trick.

After that, things got *really* silly.

The paramedics, naturally enough, wanted to get Strug off to hospital to have her ankle X-rayed. But there was no way the gymnast was going to miss the medals ceremony, even with her ankle in a makeshift plaster. So her coach – with the sheepish air of a father taking a toddler to bed clutching her teddy bear – carried her to the podium in his arms. The TV commentator did his stuff: '. . . an inspiration to every youngster, or every adult, who has ever had a dream . . .' And by that time, if you were not blubbing your eyes out as the Stars and Stripes were hoisted, there was something wrong with you.

It was one of those magical, embarrassing, no-holds-barred, irony-free moments in which Uncle Sam revels.

And all because of a sprained ankle.

When Strug finally got to hospital, she was diagnosed with a third-degree lateral sprain and tendon damage. The injury was nothing major, but enough to keep her out of the rest of the games and end her hopes of adding an individual medal to team gold.

But she had done enough. Enough to get the Olympic gold she had craved since she was a small girl. Enough to secure her immortality. Enough to win a place in the hearts of her fellow Americans. Enough to justify the hard work and the savage diets and the 24/7 training regimes that are the lot of a top-flight athlete.

'I sacrificed my childhood for gymnastics,' Strug once said in an interview. She was only thirteen when she left her family home in Tucson for Bela Karolyi's training camp in Houston; fourteen when she competed at the Barcelona Olympics. She would not be eligible today. A minimum age of sixteen has been introduced at the Olympics – a response, partly, to the pressures to which young girls like Kerri Strug used to be exposed.

After the inevitable whirl of publicity following Atlanta – the chat-show appearances, the visits to the White House, the deification on the back of a cereal packet – Strug went to college in California, then moved to Washington, where she was offered a job in the Justice Department, touring the country giving motivational talks to at-risk youngsters. She still runs marathons, but has turned her back on gymnastics. The teenager with short-cropped hair has become a glamorous long-haired blonde in a business suit.

'People still come up to me in the street and tell me I look familiar,' she said in a recent interview. 'They ask, "Were we at high school together?" or "Do you go to my church?" When I say I was a gymnast, everything falls into place.'

Of her Atlanta heroics, she says modestly: 'I wasn't the tiger. I was the cat who was always there and came back.'

Bobby Baun: 'The Best Break I Ever Had'

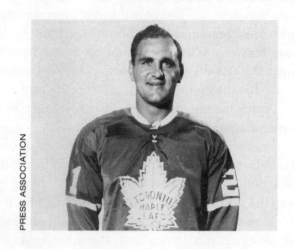

Sportsmen, as a species, are the most competitive human beings on the planet. Long after the match is over, they are still arguing about who should have won, who played a blinder, who cheated, who had the rub of the green.

And nothing gets them bickering more than a good barney about the relative seriousness of different injuries.

If Kerri Strug ever met Canadian ice hockey player Bobby Baun at a party, the conversation would go something like this:

Baun: Well, whaddya know? Kerri Strug! The girl who sprained her ankle in Atlanta!

Strug: That's the one.

Baun: Did it hurt real bad, Kerri?

Strug: You betcha, Bob. The pain was, like,
        awesome. I was crying like a baby.
Baun: Crying, huh?
Strug: Yep.
Baun: Sprained ankle, huh?
Strug: Yep.
Baun: Awesome, huh?
Strug: Yep.
Baun: Well, I *broke* my ankle. Still played on. Didn't
        whine. Never showed a living soul how much
        I was hurting. Jus' went about my business.
        No squealing. And you wanna know
        something, Kerri? I didn't need no goddam
        Hungarian coach to carry me around after the
        game. I jus' walked normal. Then I played in
        the next match, as if nothing had happened.
        Sprained ankle? Ha! You kids today jus' don't
        know . . .

Bobby Baun, originally from Saskatchewan, played for the
Toronto Maple Leafs in the early 1960s. He was chunkily
built, judging by the old black-and-white TV footage, and
not particularly mobile: better at getting in the way of the
opposition than performing feats of brilliance of his own. A
squad player. A journeyman. A hockey jock from the old
school. There is nothing in his career stats to catch the eye
of posterity. He was just a solid, hard-working pro, earning
his living in an age of sporting innocence.

  Modern ice hockey players wear protective helmets, like
batsmen in cricket, which makes them indistinguishable to
the spectator. Baun, playing in less squeamish times, seems
three-dimensional in comparison: a creature of flesh and
blood, from his bulldog jaw to the slight bald patch on the

top of his head. Even from the fuzzy TV images, you feel you know the man. There is something reassuringly primitive about him. You can imagine him stomping around Saskatchewan in Neanderthal times, coming home to his cave with half a dead bison slung over a shoulder.

His fifteen minutes of sporting fame came in the 1964 Stanley Cup, the ice hockey equivalent of the end-of-season World Series in baseball. The Maple Leafs faced the Detroit Red Wings in the best-of-seven series and were trailing 2-3 by the time of the sixth game, which was played in Detroit – a crunch match, in other words, one that the Maple Leafs had to win to keep their title hopes alive.

Midway through the match, Baun was involved in a goalmouth collision with a Detroit player. After a lengthy stoppage, he was carried off on a stretcher, with strapping around his ankle. It was obviously a serious injury, a fracture by the look of it, and it seemed inevitable that he would take no further part in the match. Ice hockey is a contact sport, one of the roughest of all, and there was no way anyone would risk a broken ankle . . .

Bobby Baun had other ideas. He had the uncomplicated up-and-at-'em outlook of sportsmen of his generation. Unless you were dead, you played. Your team needed you. You had no choice.

And this was the Stanley Cup, the biggest prize in ice hockey.

'They took me to the infirmary,' he remembers, 'and the guys who looked at it didn't think I could hurt it any more than I already had, so they froze it and I went back to play the game. I knew it was broken: I didn't need any X-rays to tell me that. But I didn't want to miss extra time. I told the trainer he had to do everything possible to get me out there.

He gave me a shot of painkiller, which numbed the ankle, and taped it tight. Then I laced up my skate and went back to the bench.'

As the game went into extra time, with the teams deadlocked, Baun returned to the ice. There was so much strapping around his foot that it was a wonder he could walk, never mind keep his balance, with only the thin blade of the skate to support his ankle. Spectators winced every time he made a tackle. It seemed only a matter of time before he would have to be stretchered off again.

Instead – deliciously – the injured player scored the winning goal. Baun was normally a stolid defender, who seldom ventured out of his own half, but now he struck a speculative thirty-yard shot that deflected off a defender and into the back of the net. Pandemonium. Hoopla! Slaps on the back for Baun. The Maple Leafs had tied the series 3-3 and lived to fight another day.

Everything now depended on the final game – at which Baun, perforce, would be a spectator. As soon as X-rays revealed that he had broken his ankle, he would be out of the game for six weeks minimum, walking around on crutches with his foot in plaster. Yes?

No. Baun was not a fool. He knew that an X-ray would give the game away in seconds. So he simply refused to let the club doctors examine him. Two days later he was back on the ice, doing his bit for the team, which won the game 4-0, taking the Stanley Cup for the third season in a row.

'It was the best break I ever had,' Baun joked, when the secret finally came to light.

After the heroics of 1964, his later career was frustratingly patchy. One disappointment followed another. He agitated for better pay and conditions, which soured his relationship with his manager, Punch Imlach. In the 1966–67 season, he broke his toe, and was mainly a spectator when the Maple Leafs won the Stanley Cup again. Baun refused to take part in the celebrations. After that, he became a gypsy of his sport, a fading star, unsettled wherever he went. In little more than three years, he moved from the Oakland Seals to the Detroit Red Wings to the Buffalo Sabres to the St Louis Blues, before being traded back to the Maple Leafs, where he enjoyed a brief renaissance. But a neck injury early in the 1972–73 season ended his NHL career at the age of thirty-six.

Baun ran a cattle farm for a time and was then tempted into management, coaching the Toronto Toros during the 1975–76 season. When they performed abjectly, finishing bottom of the league, he was out of a job. He went back to the farm, then had a spell selling insurance. In the 1980s, back on his old hobbyhorse, Baun organised an NHL alumni association and campaigned for a better pension deal. His own pension, after seventeen seasons in the NHL, was a paltry $7622 a year.

The hero of the 1964 Stanley Cup is now in his mid-seventies. That glorious evening – when pain and pleasure dissolved into each other – must seem a lifetime away. But if Baun the hockey player never scaled those heights again, it is worth recording one episode from his later life when he demonstrated sporting courage of the highest order.

The Toronto Toros, the team he managed for a season, once performed so shambolically against Cleveland that they threw away an 8-2 lead and lost the match 10-9. Baun, incandescent, fined every member of the team $500. The fines were later rescinded, after a storm of protest in the locker room, but any fan who has ever followed any sport will understand exactly where Baun was coming from, and cheer him to the echo.

There can sometimes be as much courage in challenging player power – reminding mollycoddled professional sportsmen of their duty to give 100 per cent effort at all times – as in playing hockey with a broken ankle.

Graham Mourie: 'My Father Thought I Was Being a Bit Unwise'

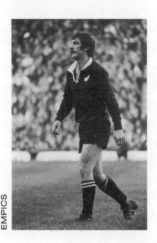

EMPICS

From broken necks to sprained and fractured ankles, and just about every part of the body in between, physical injuries and the courage to overcome them have provided some of the most stirring stories in sport. Many feature in this book. But courage is not primarily a physical attribute, the ability to cope with pain. It is a state of mind.

Some people are born brave: you see it in the set of their jaw, the glint of steel in their eyes. Others are naturally timid, skittish, like nervous animals. But it is an arena of human observation where first appearances can be more than usually deceptive. It is the little old lady with the mousy manner who tackles the burglar, the twenty-stone bruiser who keels over in a faint in the dentist's waiting-room. Circumstances change people. Crises bring out unsuspected qualities, both good and bad. Nothing in the human comedy stands still.

Ask a friend what is the most courageous thing they have done in their life, and their answer, once they have had time to ponder the question, will probably surprise you. They will not choose something obviously heroic – running into a burning house to save a child – but something less dramatic. The courage to change jobs. Or to end a relationship. Or to reveal an embarrassing secret. Or to stick by a friend. Some little crossroads in their life when they had a choice, and agonised over that choice, and upset other people with the decision they made.

New Zealand rugby captain Graham Mourie certainly upset a few people with the choice he made in 1981. It seems obvious now, a decision that any decent man would have taken. It was not so obvious at the time. Friends berated him. Strangers abused him. Hate mail plopped on to his doormat. Mourie had taken a stand and he paid a price for it – the heaviest price of all if you are a New Zealand rugby player, in a country where rugby is a religion.

He had given up the captaincy of his beloved All Blacks, spurned the opportunity to lead out his country against its greatest rival, the Springboks. In a nutshell, he had refused, when his team-mates had not refused, to play against the South Africa of the apartheid era.

The story of the struggle against apartheid, and of the role played in that struggle by sport, has been told many times. It is a story of heroes and villains, sometimes of heroes who were not quite so heroic as they seemed and sometimes of villains who were not quite so villainous. The essentials of

the plot may have been black and white, but there were
many shades of grey in the middle, particularly in New
Zealand, where the issues were always hotly debated, without producing a lasting consensus.

In the 1950s, when the All Blacks toured South Africa,
the New Zealand Rugby Union (NZRU) effectively col-
luded with the racist policies of their hosts, with Maori
players not considered for selection. By the end of the
1960s, as protests against apartheid spread across the sporting world, such a policy became unsustainable. In 1973
the Labour government led by Norman Kirk cancelled a
scheduled Springbok tour of New Zealand. The NZRU
protested about the involvement of politics in sport, but
seemed to have lost the argument. South Africa had become
an international pariah, her sports teams shunned world-
wide. Only the election of the ultra-conservative Robert
Muldoon as prime minister in 1976 altered the political
equation.

Muldoon, the darling of voters in redneck rural commu-
nities, sanctioned an All Black tour to South Africa in 1976,
causing such an international furore that twenty-five
African nations boycotted the Montreal Olympics in
protest. Muldoon was mulishly unrepentant. Ignoring the
1977 Gleneagles Agreement, under which Commonwealth
countries resolved to discourage sporting contacts with
South Africa, he gave his blessing to a Springbok tour of
New Zealand in 1981. It was an election year, and he knew
his constituency.

All hell broke loose when the tour was announced. The
Australian prime minister Malcolm Fraser was so disgusted
that he refused permission for the plane carrying the South
African team to refuel in Australia. Anti-apartheid protest-
ers in New Zealand vowed to disrupt the tour at every

opportunity. But Muldoon and the NZRU – backed, it must be said, by large swathes of the rugby-mad New Zealand public – dug in their heels. As far as they were concerned, it was business as usual.

The All Black captain did not, could not, support that line.

Born of farming stock, Graham Mourie was far from being an instinctive liberal. In many ways, he had the values of an old-style conservative. When he later became a father, his parenting methods were touchingly rudimentary: he would offer his children rewards if they got to the age of sixteen without having tattoos or body piercings; further rewards if they reached twenty-one without having smoked. He was a simple, unpretentious, plain-talking man. But even a simple man could not blind himself to the evils of apartheid.

'I have always had a problem with being honest with myself in affairs of conscience,' he says, with touching modesty. *He* had a problem? What about the head-in-the-sand brigade running New Zealand rugby, pretending that what happened in South Africa was none of their business?

Mourie – who had not been on the 1976 tour of South Africa – had read books about the country, talked to people who had been there, studied the political fall-out in other countries where the Springboks had toured. Everything pointed in the same direction. Others could do what they wanted. He, Graham Mourie, had to follow his conscience and boycott the tour.

'I think one of the issues in our society is that we are generally hedonistic,' he explained, years later. 'We do what will make us feel good rather than what we know is right.'

If ordinary New Zealanders seemed unwilling to engage with questions of ethics and morality, the government of

Robert Muldoon was still shamelessly using the tour to make electoral capital. Keep politics out of sport! It was a facile slogan, but shout it from the rooftops and it made a potent rallying cry.

Feelings were running high and, after Mourie had announced his withdrawal from the team, he received far more brickbats than bouquets.

Today, he is able to laugh off the brickbats, make light of the hate mail, play down the rancour. 'My father and members of my family thought I was being a bit unwise,' he says. A bit? You can bet some much stronger language than that was deployed chez Mourie in 1981. But how can you not admire his calmness under fire? To the courage to say no can be added the courage to say no in a firm, but non-acrimonious way.

'I don't think you lose friends over that sort of thing,' he says. 'You might lose acquaintances.'

Among his All Black team-mates, the reaction was mixed. Some would have liked to follow his lead, according to Mourie, but did not feel they could do so without jeopardising their international futures. Others felt let down by their captain. Mark Donaldson, in particular, made no bones of his feelings. He was furious at Mourie and stated publicly that he should not be picked for New Zealand again. The battle lines were drawn.

Mourie won the battle hands down. The tour went ahead, but against such a backdrop of violent protest, unprecedented in New Zealand history, that even many of the rugby diehards came to recognise that it should never have taken place. What meaningful sporting contest was possible in such an atmosphere of bitterness?

When the match in Hamilton was abandoned, after fans invaded the pitch, the news reverberated around the world.

'It was like the sun coming up,' remembers Nelson Mandela, who heard of the abandonment in his prison cell on Robben Island. The good guys were pushing the bad guys back, like forwards in a rolling maul. And Mourie, demonstrably, was on the side of the good guys. Instead of becoming an outcast, he was welcomed back into the All Black fold later in the same year, when he was selected as captain for the tour of Romania and France.

But at the time, lest we forget, there was nothing inevitable about his victory. He had to take the flak, put his whole playing career at risk. While others dithered, he led from the front.

'Leadership doesn't necessarily imply being popular,' Mourie once said in an interview. 'Leadership is making the right decisions.'

In 1981, as his country tore itself apart, the New Zealand captain did exactly that.

Wayne Shelford: The Battle of Nantes

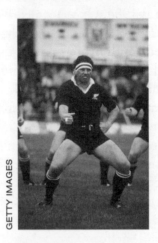

GETTY IMAGES

Courage, like beauty, can be fiendishly hard to calibrate. If one takes Graham Mourie as the benchmark by which other All Black players should be judged, then Wayne Shelford would not get a gallantry medal, but a dishonourable discharge. Where Mourie led by shining example, Shelford failed to follow.

All that can be said in Shelford's defence is that he was not alone. He ran with the pack. Most of us do.

By the mid-1980s, post-Mourie, when opposition to apartheid had forced South Africa into the sporting wilderness, there were still quite a few sportsmen dotted around the world who refused to toe the party line. There was a trickle of rebel cricket tours to South Africa. Principles became more elastic when South African sponsors opened the chequebooks. And the rugby world was even more myopic.

South Africa – incredibly, with hindsight – remained a full member of the International Rugby Board throughout the apartheid era. An official England tour of South Africa took place as late as 1984. Only one member of that squad, Ralph Knibbs of Bristol, withdrew on grounds of principle. Ireland also toured South Africa in the 1980s. It felt like the rest of the world had woken up, while rugby players still had their heads down in the scrum.

Of all the countries reluctant to sever sporting links with South Africa, none was more obdurate than New Zealand. The NZRU only cancelled a planned tour of South Africa in 1986 with extreme reluctance, after losing a court case. That seemed to be the end of the matter. But the rank-and-file All Black players, to their shame, voted with their feet.

Of the original thirty-strong tour party, which included the young Wayne Shelford, twenty-eight toured South Africa anyway. They called themselves the Cavaliers, were handsomely paid, despite being technically amateurs, and in terms of their long-term careers, escaped with relative impunity: they received a mere two-match ban and were then welcomed back into the All Black fold.

Shelford emerged without credit from this grubby episode. Young though he was, he could have taken a stand, refused to take South African money, and followed the example of Graham Mourie. All it took was a little courage . . . But it would be hard on the Rotorua-born forward to deny him a place in a book about sporting bravery. Morally, he may have been a mouse. Physically, he was a lion.

Just months after his return from South Africa, Shelford took centre stage in one of the most bruising encounters in sporting history. It was ostensibly a rugby international between France and New Zealand, played on 15 November 1986. It has been known ever since as the Battle of Nantes. Suddenly sport was not mimicking war. It *was* war.

New Zealand had won the first Test in the series 19-7, which was a red rag to the raging bull that was French rugby. 'There is lot of passion in our game, perhaps too much,' the French player Raphael Ibanez once conceded. 'You could call the passion a craziness, a madness. One of the reasons rugby is so popular in the south of France is that it allows people to express themselves.' Express themselves? Can't they just sip cognac, entertain their mistresses and play boules in the town square?

At Nantes, hell-bent on revenge for defeat in the first match, the French forwards expressed themselves so vigorously that, by twenty minutes into the match, Wayne Shelford, nicknamed 'Buck' because of the prominence of his front teeth, had lost three of those teeth after being kicked in the face in a ruck. He was still spitting out fragments of teeth when he found himself at the bottom of a second ruck, grimly trying to hold on to the ball. 'I am not quite sure what happened after that,' he admits. 'I was in la-la land from then on.' Everything happened in such a violent blur that it was like a drive-by shooting.

As Shelford held on to the ball, the French hooker, Daniel Dubroca, tried to kick it out of his hands, but only succeeded in catching him in the groin, raking his studs across the All Black's scrotum. 'It bloody well hurt,' says Shelford, who remembers that bit perfectly. 'I just chucked the old proverbial Jesus water down my shorts to make it feel better. That didn't do a lot, so we just played on.' He was still feeling groggy when, at the next ruck, another French forward, Jean-Pierre Garuet, flew in from the side and knocked him out cold. This time the All Black did accept that he needed treatment and staggered to the side of the pitch, where he was examined by the team physio, with a French cameraman in close attendance.

At this point in the story, in that kindly parallel universe beyond sport, sanity would have prevailed. The wounded New Zealand player would have left the scene, to sympathetic French applause, and been taken to the nearest hospital in an ambulance. Doctors would have examined him, operated under anaesthetic and prescribed a period of complete rest. One likes to think of the patient, a week later, sitting gingerly up in bed, nibbling grapes and bantering with French nurses.

But, by now, the Battle of Nantes was following its own bloody logic.

The New Zealand physio pulled down Shelford's shorts, saw that his scrotum was badly ripped, with one testicle hanging out, and in an operation beamed by television into French living-rooms, stitched up the wound. Shelford, who has no memory of his heroics, stumbled back on to the pitch, played doggedly on, and was not substituted until twenty minutes from time. Even then, he refused treatment, and just sat quietly on the bench with his team-mates. The full extent of the wound impinged on his consciousness only in the dressing-room afterwards. It would require more than twenty stitches.

France, uncompromising to the end, went on to win the match 16-3. But who now remembers the score? They only remember the madman from New Zealand who insisted on playing on with his testicle dangling out.

It was, in its way, the *ne plus ultra* of manliness in sport. Any athlete, of either sex, can sprain an ankle, break a collarbone, rupture a hernia. But in the roll-call of sporting courage, the New Zealander holds a unique place, revered by his sex. In a roughhouse sport, it was the most X-rated moment of all.

Shelford's subsequent playing career was short but sweet. The Battle of Nantes was the last Test match he lost – as he wryly put it, an isolated '*faux pas*'. Part of the New Zealand team that won the 1987 World Cup, he took over as captain, in a side that carried all before it. Shelford was a superb leader on the field, but also found the time to institute improvements to the famous pre-match 'haka', taking his team-mates to a Maori school to learn the 'Ka Mate' dance that players still use to this day.

When he was dropped from the team in 1990, to make way for Zinzan Brooke, there was general disbelief that such an inspirational leader should have been sidelined when still the right side of thirty. Fans brought 'Bring Back Buck' banners to matches in protest.

Shelford coached for a time in Britain, including a spell at Saracens, before returning to New Zealand. In June 2007, with the same matter-of-fact courage he had shown at the Battle of Nantes, more than twenty years before, he revealed that he was receiving treatment for cancer and asked for his privacy to be respected as he focused on recovery.

A fresh challenge now faced the former All Black captain. It could be taken for granted that he would meet it with resolve, and unquenchable bravery.

Andy Flower, Henry Olonga and Those Armbands

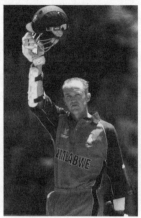

If the apartheid regime in South Africa divided the sporting world, setting team-mate against team-mate, the regime of Robert Mugabe polarised opinion just as starkly – and still does.

The frenzied buck-passing that preceded the 2003 Cricket World Cup, co-hosted by South Africa and Zimbabwe, left a sour taste that still lingers. The British government wanted the England team to refuse to play against Zimbabwe in Harare, but was not willing to underwrite the costs of their withdrawal. The ECB dithered, the ICC stuck its head in the sand, and the England players, captained by Nasser Hussein, were caught in the middle. Eventually, ingloriously, they refused to play Zimbabwe on security grounds, rather than political grounds, and forfeited the match. The Australians, even more ingloriously, had no qualms about playing in Zimbabwe, and no problem beating their hosts by seven wickets – not that anyone was taking much notice of the cricket any more.

In the morass of humbug, a protest by two men – Zimbabwean cricketers Andy Flower and Henry Olonga – stood out like a beacon of integrity, casting its beams all around the world. Where the administrators had tied themselves in knots, and the politicians prevaricated, the players cut to the chase, with the authority of their anger.

And the world – finally – sat up and took notice.

Andy Flower, the senior of the two players, at the time of writing the England cricket coach, made the initial running. Born in 1968, Flower was old enough to remember the birth of Zimbabwe, its emergence as an independent nation, and the tidal wave of optimism on which Robert Mugabe had been swept to power. 'I had an idyllic upbringing,' he once told an interviewer. But despite his success on the cricket field, where he became the leading batsman in Zimbabwean history, Flower could not blind himself to the violence and intimidation that were slowly engulfing his country.

Things came to a head in early 2003, shortly before the scheduled start of the World Cup. First a close friend of Flower was evicted from his farm, joined the Movement for Democratic Change, but found himself threatened with arrest and imprisonment. Then a leading opposition MP, Job Sikhala, was subjected to brutal torture in prison. It was too much for Flower, who put in a phone call to Henry Olonga, one of his Zimbabwe team-mates. The two men met in Harare, where Flower got straight to the point. 'I think someone needs to take a stand. And I think that person is you.'

He chose Olonga for two reasons. First, because he was black and Flower was white: between them, they could speak with an authority that neither on his own could muster. Second, because Olonga was a talented young cricketer whose sphere of influence extended beyond cricket – he had just had a surprise hit as a singer. If a popular public figure like Henry Olonga could be persuaded to denounce the Mugabe regime, people really would start listening.

Olonga, like Flower, has good memories of the early years under Mugabe. 'I thought he was a very fair, true, honest President,' he recalls. But two years before he met Flower, he had been handed a dossier of human rights abuses that could not be ignored. The more he examined the evidence, the more determined he became to take a stance. Among the role models who inspired him was Maximus, the character played by Russell Crowe in *Gladiator*, a movie he watched again and again. 'I wanted to be the slave who defied an emperor.'

What to do? Flower felt that pulling out of the tournament altogether would not have been fair on the younger Zimbabwe players at the start of their careers. So they hatched Plan B. At the start of the opening game, against Namibia, both players would wear black armbands. They would then issue a statement mourning the death of democracy in Zimbabwe. And take the consequences.

After they unveiled the plan to their team-mates on the morning of the match, the mood in the dressing-room was electric. 'The poo hit the fan,' Olonga remembers.

'Do you realise the consequences?' gasped Vince Hogg, head of the Zimbabwe Cricket Union.

The honest answer would have been: no, they did not; they could only guess at the consequences; hit and hope, like tail-end batsmen. But the die had been cast. The world had seen their black armbands. And the world was now digesting the statement they had drafted.

'In wearing a black armband . . . we are mourning the death of democracy in our beloved Zimbabwe . . . making a silent plea to those responsible to stop the abuse of human rights in Zimbabwe. In doing so, we pray that our small action may help to restore sanity and dignity to our nation.'

Simple. Clear. Word-perfect. Suddenly the result of a cricket match did not matter a damn. But if there had been no cricket match, would anyone have been watching? Great actors need a great stage.

Beyond taking a courageous public stand, what did Andy Flower and Henry Olonga actually achieve in 2003? It is impossible to say. The wheels of history turn so slowly sometimes that you can hardly see them move.

The day after their protest, the cricketing circus moved on. Shane Warne, sensationally, was found to have used a banned diuretic, tried to blame his mother, and was sent home from the World Cup in disgrace. By the time the press had gorged their fill on that story, the black armbands were largely forgotten.

But not totally forgotten. Not by Robert Mugabe and his henchmen.

For Flower and Olonga, marked men as far as the Zimbabwean authorities were concerned, an uncertain future awaited, fraught with danger. 'It was scary and emotional because we worried about the repercussions,' Flower remembers. 'But along with the scary feeling was a real sense of being alive.'

Flower and his family – including his heavily pregnant wife – had made plans for a mass exodus as soon as the tournament was over. Olonga was less well prepared. With time running out, as soon as Zimbabwe were eliminated from the tournament, he could expect swift and savage reprisals. Providentially, the weather intervened.

In the normal run of things, the three words cricketers most hate are 'rain stopped play'. But the rain that washed out Zimbabwe's group match against Pakistan was a lifeline for Olonga. The wash-out meant that Zimbabwe went through to the next stages in South Africa. He travelled to the matches with the rest of the team then, after the last game, in East London, announced his retirement from international cricket.

Back in Zimbabwe, a warrant had been issued for his arrest on a treason charge, which carried the death penalty. But Olonga was not going back to Zimbabwe. He had made good his escape.

'We didn't change anything, and weren't strong enough to do so,' said Flower later. 'But we got an amazing response from people who felt they had been jogged out of their apathy.'

Henry Olonga echoes these sentiments. 'Did I change the world? Probably not. Did I change Zimbabwe? Probably not. But I played my part. If I hadn't embraced the moment, I could have been a nobody, had a mediocre World Cup, and nobody would have remembered. Now I'm remembered as the man who wore a black armband.'

Tom Molineaux: Black Ajax

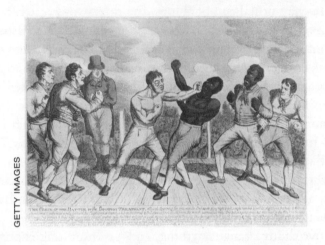

Flower and Olonga's defiance of the Mugabe regime was a reminder that even in the twenty-first century, sport can still be a dangerous arena, where lives as well as limbs are put at risk.

Modern sportsmen, as a rule, are protected against life-threatening injuries. And so they should be. Sport is meant to be fun. There is no fun in seeing corpses strewn across a playing field. But that same safety-first culture narrows the window of opportunity for physical courage. The heroes have shrunk.

Take motor racing. Safety improvements to cars have meant that fatalities are now extremely rare. The sport has advanced, put its house in order, weeded out unacceptable risks, discharged its duty of care to drivers; in short, become a more gentle pursuit. But something of real human worth has been lost in the progress. The winning driver in a Grand Prix is simply the one who has driven fastest. He is not, as he would once have been, a man who had to take hair-raising, death-defying risks to beat his rivals.

To wax nostalgic about the days when sport involved extreme physical danger would be absurd. But in a book about sporting courage, it would be remiss to neglect the Dark Ages of sport, when no quarter was given, when there were no ambulances on stand-by, and when the likes of Tom Molineaux, 'Black Ajax', inflamed the public imagination with their bravery.

I first encountered Black Ajax – one of the superstars of bare-knuckle boxing in the Regency era – through the novel of the same name by the late George MacDonald Fraser. I had never taken much interest in nineteenth-century boxing, so the name of Tom Molineaux was new to me. But in the hands of a literary master, the untutored ex-slave from America who took on the great Tom Cribb, unde-feated Champion of England, springs four-square from the page.

This is not chocolate-box history – sentimental, sani-tised – but something rawer: a re-creation of an age when masculinity was defined in frighteningly primitive terms. 'Boxing is a barbarous sport,' said Fraser, when I questioned him about his novel. 'It really ought to be banned. There is no excuse for it in a civilised society. And yet . . .' His voice tailed off and, for a second, he was back in that rough, uncomplicated, manly world, where boxers fought to a standstill and, amid the blood and the gore and the baying crowds, there was a flickering nobility.

Molineaux, the prototype of the great black heavyweights who have dominated the sport ever since, was born in 1784 to parents enslaved by a wealthy Virginian plantation-owner.

Because of his size and strength, he was selected to take part in fights with slaves from neighbouring estates – a common practice at the time. The planters used to wager large sums on the outcome of the fights, and Molineaux soon made his owner a wealthy man. The owner showed his appreciation by granting the slave his freedom, whereupon Molineaux sailed to England, hoping to earn a living as a professional boxer.

It was a brave decision, a journey into the unknown. In his 1867 classic *Pugilistica: A History of English Boxing*, Henry Downes Miles writes admiringly of the courage shown by the American: 'Unnoticed, unheralded, unfriended and unknown, this sable gladiator made his way to London.'

Technically, Molineaux was still quite a crude performer, but under the tutelage of Bill Richmond, another former slave, he became a formidable fighter, one of the toughest in the business. Away from the ring, he was a voracious womaniser and already starting to fall prey to the alcoholism that would later destroy him. As Downes Miles delicately puts it: 'He devoted himself by turns to Bacchus and Venus.' But Regency boxing fans – the Fancy, as they were known – flocked to see this strong, muscular black man who seemed able to take punch after punch without protest.

Molineaux saw off all-comers until there was a clamour for him to take on Tom Cribb. The English champion, past thirty, was contemplating retirement, but with everyone licking their lips at the prospect of a Cribb–Molineaux showdown, a fight duly took place at Copthorne Gap, near East Grinstead, on 18 December 1810. In filthy weather nearly ten thousand spectators tramped for miles through the mud to see it.

There is a contemporary account of the fight in Pierce

Egan's *Boxiana* and, even at this remove of time, the courage shown by both men, fifty years before the Marquess of Queensberry rules were introduced, is mind-boggling.

Boxers in the Regency period fought not only with bare fists, but until one of them quit or was rendered unconscious. There was no limit on the duration or number of rounds, which would end when one fighter was knocked down. The next would begin after a thirty-second break. Kicking, biting and gouging were not allowed, but otherwise it was each man for himself – until one of them, literally, collapsed.

The Cribb–Molineaux fight lasted a stupefying thirty-nine rounds. Through the fog of Egan's breathless Regency slang ('Cribb exhibited the first signs of claret . . . The Black rallied in fine twig . . . left-handed hits planted on his nob . . . but Cribb knocked him down, his peeper materially damaged . . .'), one can glimpse a truly colossal sporting encounter.

As early as round two, Cribb's mouth was bleeding. In round three, Molineaux took a vicious right to the ribs. Round six saw Cribb subside to the ground. In round seven, it was the American's turn, floored by a haymaker to the side of the head. By round twelve, the two men were slugging it out for all they were worth, trading blows to the head and body. In round fifteen, Molineaux was knocked out by a punch to the throat. In the next round, he went down, exhausted. By round nineteen, he had rallied and was meting out massive punishment himself. Cribb fell, seemingly unconscious, then fought back hard, landing a heavy blow to Molineaux's left eye. By round twenty-six, the eye had closed completely, and the American was staggering about the ring in confusion. In the following round, the two boxers were so exhausted that they leaned on each other until they both fell. Then . . .

What happened next is one of the great talking points in early boxing, impossible now to resolve. The Englishman was unable to come out for the twenty-ninth round, having taken heavy punishment. His seconds stepped in and accused Molineaux of holding pistol balls in his hands to increase his punching power. A row ensued, which gave Cribb time to clear his head. It sounds like a delaying tactic, like the later famous piece of shenanigans in the fight between Henry Cooper and Cassius Clay in 1963, when the American was in trouble and his trainer, Angelo Dundee, caused a delay in proceedings by making a nick in his glove.

Whatever the rights and wrongs of the row, Molineaux ended up on the losing side. 'Me no can fight no more,' he protested, punch-drunk, at the start of the thirty-ninth round. He was persuaded to go into the ring one last time, but collapsed unconscious within seconds.

His defeat was wreathed in more nobility than a hundred victories. 'Molineaux in this context proved himself as courageous a man as ever an adversary contended with,' writes Downes Miles. Three days after the fight, through his seconds, Molineaux wrote to Cribb challenging him to a rematch. Truculent, irrepressible, defiant in defeat, the American hinted that, if the weather had been better, he would have won the first fight. He even had the temerity, in the nicest possible way, to play the race card. 'I cannot omit the opportunity of expressing a confident hope that the circumstances of my being of a different colour . . . will not in any way operate to my prejudice.' Like great boxers through the ages, he was down but not out: he had lived to fight another day.

The rematch the following year attracted even bigger crowds than the first fight, but ended in anticlimax: Cribb won with comparative ease, after just nineteen rounds. Five years later, Tom Molineaux was dead. His alcoholic excesses caught up with him, and he died in a barn in Galway, having been taken in by two black soldiers who took pity on him.

Yet his name lingers faintly on: a byword for physical endurance in the face of punishment. If bare-knuckle boxing belongs to history, it is not a chapter in sporting history that one should read with revulsion and nothing but revulsion. To their Regency contemporaries, the great boxers of the day were 'actors on a stage of valour', fitting role models for the young men who might be called to serve their country in the Napoleonic wars. Or, as Pierce Egan put it, in his hifalutin but still eloquent way: 'Pugilism . . . taught men to admire true courage . . . acquire notions of honour . . . and invincibility of soul'.

In an age when sportsmen were as much warriors as celebrities, Black Ajax epitomised that spirit of invincibility.

The Death Match

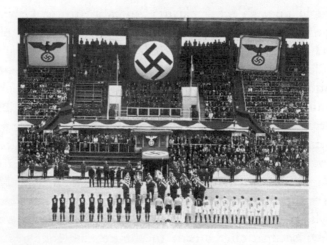

If boxers put their lives on the line, footballers generally risk nothing worse than a broken leg. To the cynical public, they are the biggest wimps in sport, writhing in pain after falling over in the penalty area.

It was not always thus. I have already reprised the famous story of Bert Trautmann and his broken neck. To a man who had fought in the war, such heroics were instinctive, even natural – unimaginable today. The same could be said of one of the most gruesomely celebrated of all football matches: the Death Match, played in Kiev on 9 August 1942, when a local Ukrainian team had the temerity to beat a crack German XI, and paid with their lives.

The match is steeped in so much mythology and counter-mythology – not to mention being bowdlerised by Hollywood in the awful *Escape to Victory*, starring Michael

Caine, Pele and Sylvester Stallone – that it is difficult to put it in accurate perspective. During the Soviet era, the story of the match was virtually airbrushed out of history. It had embarrassing as well as heroic elements. What were the Ukrainians doing playing football with the Nazis in the first place? They certainly did not have the blessing of the Communist Party. In fact, they were dangerously independent-minded, and probably bourgeois revisionists with it. But thanks to books like the excellent *Dynamo* by Andy Dougan, a good deal of the fog of history has now cleared, leaving a cast of authentic, if ghostly, heroes who were a credit to their country and to their sport.

FC Start had their origins in a Kiev bakery, where a number of former Dynamo Kiev players, notably the goalkeeper Nikolai Trusevich, found themselves working during the Nazi occupation. Outside the bakery, life for ordinary Ukrainians was harrowing and precarious. The spectre of death hung over the city. By November 1941, an estimated hundred thousand Ukrainians, including seventy-five thousand Jews, had been murdered. Even inside the bakery, under conditions of forced labour, where twenty-four-hour shifts were the norm, nobody was safe. In one infamous incident, twenty-two workers were shot after someone threw broken glass into a batch of bread.

   To want to play football in such circumstances probably seems the height of frivolity today. But sport has always been a potent symbol of the normality to which people yearn to return when war is over. In the spring of 1942, as a makeshift football league developed, Trusevich rounded up a few of his old Dynamo Kiev team-mates and assembled an eleven that could compete with the best sides in the city. FC Start were disadvantaged in umpteen ways, some trivial, some not so trivial. They were barred from training in the stadium, exhausted from their shifts in the bakery and forced to wear cut-down trousers and canvas shoes, instead of proper football kit. But nothing could stop them scoring more goals than their opponents.

In their very first match, Start beat Rukh, a team run by a Nazi collaborator, 7-2. A Hungarian garrison side was dispatched 6-2, then a team of Romanians 11-0. Their next opponents were PGS, a German military side, whom they thrashed 6-0. By this stage, Start were not just attracting enthusiastic crowds, but alarming the occupying German authorities. For the master race to be humbled by these subhuman upstarts would be a propaganda disaster. As the Start winning streak continued, the Nazis drew up active counter-measures. The bakery team had to be put in their place, and who better to do it than Flakelf, a team representing the Luftwaffe, the flower of German manhood?

The first match between FC Start and Flakelf took place on Thursday 6 August. The Ukrainians won handsomely, 5-1, despite some brutal tackles from their German opponents. The German-controlled Kiev newspapers did not even deign to report the match. The Nazi authorities ordered an immediate rematch. The irresistible force met immovable object. When would FC Start get the message and deliver the right result?

Answer: never. Deliberately losing a match goes against the deepest instincts of a sportsman. If someone had tried to exhort the same FC Start players to mutiny against the occupying Nazi regime, they would have refused: the instinct for self-preservation, in the face of certain death, would have been too strong. On the football field, in the heat of competition, a different logic applied.

Just before the match, played in the Zenit stadium, an SS

officer entered the Start dressing-room unannounced. According to Makar Goncharenko, the little winger, one of the few players to survive the war, the officer addressed the team politely in perfect Russian: 'I am the referee of today's game. I know you are a very good team. Please follow the rules, do not break any of the rules and, before the game, greet your opponents in our fashion.'

The tone may have been polite, but the message was clear. The Nazi referee expected Start to give a Nazi salute before the start of the game, as a courtesy to their opponents. The England football team had done this, to their shame, when they played a friendly against Germany in Berlin in 1938. The Foreign Office and Football Association, an unholy alliance if ever there was one, had deemed the salute advisable.

FC Start players were not so craven. Instead of giving a Nazi salute, they raised their arms, brought them back to their chests and shouted a Soviet slogan used as a battle cry by the Red Army. The die was cast.

As the game got under way, with the Nazi top brass in the grandstand, while the Start fans stood in the mud, the bias of the referee quickly became obvious. A string of brutal fouls by the Flakelf players went unpunished. Trusevich, the Start goalkeeper, was kicked in the head. There were flying elbows, shirt-pulling, scything tackles from behind. Sport had become war by other means.

The Start players were not going to shirk the challenge.

They not only won, 5-3, but humiliated their opponents. In the closing minutes, a Start player rounded the German defence, danced past the goalkeeper and, instead of scoring, kicked the ball back to the centre circle. The Nazi referee, admitting defeat, blew the final whistle before the ninety minutes were up.

Reprisals – contrary to the more lurid versions of the Death Match myth, in which the Start players were rounded up and shot straight after the match – were not immediate. In fact, FC Start played another match the following Sunday, against a Ukrainian team, and won 8-0. But the wheels of retribution had been set in motion. A few days later, the Gestapo turned up at the bakery where most of the Start players worked, arrested members of the team, took them to a secret police HQ, and interrogated them under torture. The Gestapo hoped that they would confess to being criminals or saboteurs, which would have given the Germans a pretext to execute them. None of the players cracked. One died under torture. The rest were sent to a nearby labour camp, where their prospects of survival were slim. The SS shot three of the players the following winter. Others were luckier, escaping the camp and staying hidden in Kiev until the city was liberated from German occupation in November 1943. But even their future was bleak. To their new Communist masters, the footballers were no better than Nazi collaborators. There were no happy endings in this cruellest of sporting sagas.

Today, the doomed players of FC Start seem like heroic figures, martyrs to a cause that embraced football but was also bigger than football. Perhaps that is just the hyperbole of hindsight. In 1992, fifty years after the Death Match, Goncharenko, the Start winger, and sole surviving member of the team, gave a very downbeat assessment: 'A desperate fight for survival started, which ended badly for four players. Unfortunately, they did not die because they were great footballers. They died, like many other Soviet people, because two totalitarian systems were fighting each other, and they were destined to become victims of that grand scale massacre. The death of the players is no different from many other deaths.'

Maybe so. But compared with that England football team in Berlin, giving stiff-armed Nazi salutes to order, the FC Start players were moral lions.

Eleanor Simmonds: 'In My Dream, I Only Came Second'

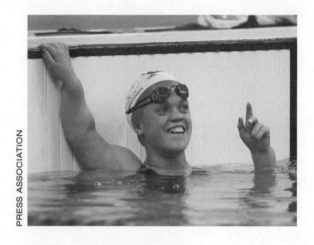

PRESS ASSOCIATION

In sport as in life, courage can take totally different forms. Is a disabled runner a role model and a disabled accountant not? I wonder.

My father, who died in 2007 at the age of eighty-two, had only one leg. He lost his other leg when he was a boy, as a result of osteomyelitis. For the rest of his life, he went around on crutches: commuting to work in the City; going for walks on Wimbledon Common; climbing stairs without protest; living as full a life as possible. I never once heard him complain.

He enjoyed televised sport, but when it came to participating, attempted nothing more strenuous than bridge. Perhaps if he had born fifty years later, he might have travelled a different journey, been lured by dreams of

Paralympic glory. Who can say? As it was, his courage, though undoubted, and inspirational, was of the passive, stoic, accepting kind – quite different from the more proactive courage of the disabled athlete.

But I would not want to deny disabled athletes their rightful place in a book about sporting courage.

And I could not possibly leave out Ellie Simmonds.

The teenage sensation of the Beijing Paralympics, Walsall-born Eleanor Simmonds has so many of the attributes of a sporting superstar that, in telling her story, it is easy to omit the most distinctive physical fact about her: she suffers from achondroplasia, or dwarfism, and stands at just three foot nine.

'I don't even think about that,' she insists. 'It's normal for me, and I've never had any problems at school or anywhere else because of my height.' Words characteristic of a doughty fighter.

She took her first swimming lesson at the age of four, competed in her first gala aged eight, and was still only nine when she watched the Athens Paralympics on television. 'That's what I want to do,' she told her mother, with all the single-minded determination of a Tiger Woods or a Lewis Hamilton. Her first sporting heroine was Nyree Lewis, a cerebral palsy sufferer who won two gold medals for Great Britain in Athens.

As attention shifted to Beijing, Ellie's parents Val and Steve decided to relocate to Swansea, so that she could join the elite group of disabled swimmers being coached by Billy Pye at the Wales National Pool. 'It takes guts to up sticks like that,' Pye reflected. 'I've got nothing but admiration for Ellie's parents for moving down here to let their daughter follow her dream.' Amen to that. How many times, behind a sporting hero or heroine, do you find equally heroic parents?

Val Simmonds, on her own admission, was homesick at first, and missed her family and friends in the Midlands. She felt the family was properly settled only when her daughter began making friends at the local comprehensive school and throwing herself into her training, swimming six days a week.

For all her talent and evident determination, Ellie Simmonds was thirteen at the time of the Beijing Olympics, and not viewed as a strong medal contender, more as a long-term prospect for the London Games in 2012. Her best chance of a medal seemed to be in the 400m freestyle, her main event, and eleven members of her family duly booked flights out to Beijing for the final. Nobody expected her to do more than make up the numbers in the 100m freestyle, held three days earlier. They underestimated – everyone underestimated – the emotional resources of one inspired, pumped-up teenager.

With twenty-five metres to go, Simmonds was beaten, second-best, out of contention. But like all great champions, she found something extra when she needed to, taking the race in an incredible final surge that brought the crowd to its feet.

'It's all a blur,' she says now. 'I just remember getting my head down, getting that last bit of energy and going for it. I was so shocked to win.'

So shocked that, after receiving her medal, she burst into tears, and looked vaguely disoriented, as if she had lost, not won. 'I had a dream about the race last night,' she told reporters. 'But in my dream I got silver.' Winning individual gold aged thirteen – the youngest British Paralympian ever to do so – had taken the girl from Walsall to an undreamed-of place.

She went on to take gold in the 400m as well, matching the double triumph of Rebecca Adlington – another British teenager catapulted to stardom by Beijing – in the main Olympics.

In physical stature, the two girls could hardly have been more different, but they endeared themselves to fans for the same reason: their essential ordinariness. Their appeal lay in their lack of glamour. They might talk wistfully of Jimmy Choo shoes or Louis Vuitton handbags, but they were rooted in the real world, in thrilling contrast to so many sporting megastars.

If Simmonds had needed raw physical determination to win her gold medals, she also showed great emotional maturity afterwards, taking time out to commiserate with Nyree Lewis, her one-time heroine, who had a disappointing Games. Back in England, when she was voted Paralympian of the Year, Simmonds did not turn up to collect her medal, for the most footling but laudable of reasons – she did not want to miss a maths class. Life got back to normal with commendable speed, with training for the 2012 Olympics given due priority.

For a time, celebrity followed her around. Her friends thought they had lost her on a visit to a shopping centre, only to find her surrounded by a crowd of well-wishers. But somehow you could tell that the plaudits would not go to her head. She had the innate modesty of the true sportswoman.

'Beijing was an amazing experience and an amazing challenge,' she said in an interview after the Games. 'I was really proud to represent my country. But I did miss my friends and family – and proper British cooking.' In an instant, you could see the frightened child behind the medal-winner: the child who had had to conquer her demons, in big ways and small.

Asked in another interview which three words best described her, she selected 'nervous', 'friendly' and 'smiley'. It was a revealing choice. We could all see the smiles, the friendliness: we missed the nervousness behind the warm, outgoing exterior.

'Being small never stopped her doing anything,' said her mother. 'There was never anything she felt she couldn't do. In her head, she is six feet tall.'

And in the hearts of her fans, a good deal taller than that.

Ben Hogan: The Wee Ice Mon

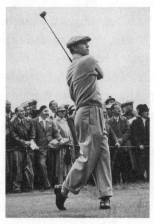

EMPICS

Every age has its own sporting heroes and moulds them in its own image. Notions of honour and manliness change from generation to generation. The currency of courage fluctuates.

David Beckham's broken metatarsal would never have captured the public imagination fifty years ago. To have made such a song and dance of such a relatively minor injury would have seemed the height of self-indulgence to the generation that had been through the war. But in the build-up to the 2002 World Cup, the fracture of a little-known bone with a sexy-sounding name made the perfect condiment to the football. It was a medical soap opera for all the family, featuring a pretty-boy hero who looked damn good on crutches. How we gorged ourselves on the unfolding drama.

When Tiger Woods won the 2008 US Open with a dodgy knee, some commentators immediately hailed it as his greatest-ever victory, the apotheosis of an extraordinary career. The sight of a golfer playing through the pain barrier, wincing after every shot, was so unfamiliar that the Battle of Wounded Knee achieved a mythic status out of all proportion to the seriousness of the injury. Even Woods himself, not normally allergic to the limelight, seemed to be embarrassed by the hype.

As the myth-making went into overdrive, and the banner headlines got ever larger, golf fans old enough to remember Ben Hogan, and the battles he went through, allowed themselves rueful smiles.

One of the paradoxical aspects of courage is that the people who furnish the most heart-warming examples of courage in action are often the coolest, least demonstrative of human beings. We respond to their hidden depths: the sense of inner battles being fought with quiet dignity.

Of all the famous sportsmen who have been likened to robots for the clinical efficiency of their play, Ben Hogan was arguably the most robotic of the lot. Everyone who saw him play envied his perfectly grooved swing. How could he eliminate so completely all the little physical kinks and gremlins that make golf such a difficult game? But Hogan's frigid personality, his almost pathological inability to smile on the golf course, was even more noteworthy.

'I play golf with friends sometimes,' Hogan once said, 'but there are never any friendly games.' The American golf writer Herbert Warren Wind recalls him playing with 'the burning frigidity of dry ice'. All the qualities that made Nick Faldo so disliked by his fellow professionals had been patented by Hogan. They made him an unnerving opponent. His great rival Sam Snead joked that the only three things he feared on a golf course were a downhill putt, lightning and Ben Hogan. When Hogan won the 1953 Open at Carnoustie, Scottish golf fans, awed by his concentration levels, nicknamed him 'The Wee Ice Mon'.

Delve into his childhood history and his manner is readily explained. Born in Dublin, Texas, in 1912, Hogan was nine when his father Chester, a blacksmith, killed himself with a shotgun – a harrowing episode that left a lifelong legacy of anxiety and sadness. A period of grinding poverty followed, and it was through earning pin-money as a caddy that Hogan first caught the golfing bug. His early years as a professional were not particularly successful, and not until Hogan was in his mid-thirties, after serving in the Army during the Second World War, did he win his first major, the 1946 PGA Championship. Further successes followed until, on 2 February 1949, came the car accident that was to define his career.

Hogan was driving through the Apache mountains in Texas, in heavy fog, when his car was involved in a head-on collision with a Greyhound bus. With his wife Valerie in the passenger seat, he threw himself across her body to protect her. Lucky he did – the steering column punctured the driver's seat and would certainly have killed him. As it was, he suffered a fractured collar bone, a double fracture of the pelvis, a left ankle fracture, broken ribs, a ruptured bladder, a deep gash by his left eye and blood-clots so serious they would cause him circulation problems for the rest of his life. It took more than an hour to free Hogan from the wreckage.

Doctors warned him he might never walk again, let alone play competitive golf. Hogan, with the single-mindedness for which he was celebrated, set about proving them wrong.

When discharged from hospital, sixty days after the

accident, he was still limping and still in pain, with his left shoulder throbbing more or less continually. Resuming the life of a full-time tour professional was not an option, so Hogan concentrated his sights on the majors and just a few other tournaments. He had always been a perfectionist on the golf course, working tirelessly to develop a swing that would hold up under pressure. Now that was put to its sternest test. It can be hard enough to hit a golf ball straight when your body is in full working order. To do it when you are having to favour one leg over the other, or when your shoulder is screaming in pain, demands superhuman self-discipline. But then self-discipline, for Hogan, had never been a problem.

It is indicative of the awe in which he was held by his contemporaries that, when he won the 1950 US Open at Merion, Pennsylvania, little more than a year after his accident, Hollywood was moved to make its first golf film, *Follow the Sun*, a cheesy biopic starring Glenn Ford as Hogan and Anne Baxter as his wife. The amiable Ford was hopelessly miscast: he missed the steel in Hogan, and if you missed the steel you missed the man. But a famous sporting victory – Hogan played with his legs in plaster and had to navigate a punishing thirty-six holes on the final day of the tournament – had passed into American folklore.

Even greater triumphs lay ahead. In 1953, his *annus mirabilis*, Hogan won three majors, a feat not previously achieved. By focusing his energies on a handful of tournaments a year, he became the pre-eminent golfer of his generation, a byword for ruthless efficiency. But, for all his dominance, rank-and-file golf fans never took him to their hearts. He was admired, but not loved. The tragically orphaned boy was too emotionally frozen to reach out for the biggest prize of all.

Even in old age, Hogan remained a cold, aloof figure, not an avuncular elder statesman in the Arnold Palmer mould. Conversationally, he was a miser, fabled for his taciturnity. When Nick Faldo, granted an audience with the great man, asked Hogan what was the secret of winning the US Open, he got a four-word answer: 'Shoot the lowest score.' Oh to have been a fly on the wall during the ensuing awkward silence.

Somewhere inside the ice man, one suspects, there was a much warmer Ben Hogan wanting to be let out. His most celebrated quotation about golf has an unexpected quality of poetry: 'As you walk down the fairway of life, you must smell the roses, for you only get to play one round.' Roses? Was this the Ben Hogan whose concentration was so intense that you could have planted a whole rose garden beside the fairway and he would not have noticed? But that other Hogan never did get out. He died in 1997, after a long battle with Alzheimer's, a loner to the end.

But who could fail to be touched by his unwavering determination? Compared with a Tiger Woods or a David Beckham, with their showmanship and their hype and their relentless PR machines, he was a model of self-effacing excellence, a stoic, a man of his times.

As his biographer Curt Sampson put it: 'Hogan had no yardage book, no golf glove, no self-congratulation, no logo, no bullshit, and no pretence. Everything he accomplished, he dug out of the ground.'

John Daly: Keeping the Show on the Road

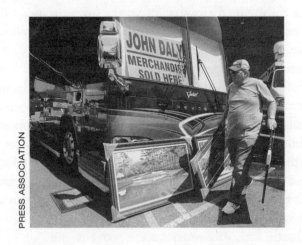

PRESS ASSOCIATION

Golfing injuries are so rare that, for all the charms of the game, it seldom serves up the kind of blood-and-guts heroics associated with the boxing ring or the rugby field. Ben Hogan was the exception that proves the rule. But that does not make golf a courage-free zone. You just need to look at the sport through a slightly different lens.

Imagine being a City banker made redundant, reduced to sleeping in the street. Would you sleep outside your old bank? Of course not. The thought of your former colleagues seeing you would be crucifying.

Or imagine being an MP chucked out by the voters, having to earn a living as a taxi driver. Would you ply your trade in Parliament Square, outside the House of Commons? Not in a million years. Your nerve would fail you.

That is why, at the level of courage, it was so moving to see John Daly at the 2009 Masters: not taking part in the tournament, but selling T-shirts and golfing memorabilia from his mobile home, parked across the street from the course. What chutzpah that took.

All the media focus at the Masters was on Tiger Woods, playing his first major after a long lay-off from injury. But in terms of sheer inspirational sporting guts, Woods was not even in the picture. It was big John Daly, the Wild Thing, one of the most manifestly, multiply flawed men in sport, who took the laurels.

Daly must have known, before he arrived at Augusta, the kind of looks he would get from golf fans. Looks of pity. Of contempt. Of derision. How dare he make a spectacle of himself outside the most hallowed venue in golf. But he was not going to hide from those looks. He was his own man, as he has always been, come rain or shine.

In John Daly's roller-coaster career, there have only really been two ups: his first major, the 1991 PGA Championship, when he won as a last-minute substitute; and the 1995 Open at St Andrews, when he beat Constantino Rocca in a play-off. Almost everything since, both on and off the course, has been down, down, down.

His problems with alcoholism have been well documented. So have his problems with gambling. And his four divorces. And his chronic weight problems. In a sport that likes to pride itself on its good manners, he has been a one-man soap opera, trashing hotel rooms, storming off golf courses, getting into trouble with the law, going into rehab, coming out of rehab, zigzagging from crisis to crisis like a golfer unable to find the fairway.

Even at times of relative success, Daly has found new ways to self-destruct. In 2005 he finished second to Tiger

Woods in the WGC-American Express tournament in San Francisco, then drove straight to Las Vegas and blew more than double his winnings on a gambling spree. Three years later, he hit rock bottom again, when he had to be locked up for a night by police in North Carolina after being found drunk and disorderly.

The USPGA responded to his latest disgrace by banning the player for six months. But, not for the first time, Daly came bouncing back. He pledged himself to compete in Europe in 2009, then surprised everyone, himself included, by finishing second in the Italian Open.

Gone, at least temporarily, was the bulging twenty-stone physique that was the outward manifestation of his chaotic lifestyle. The golfer had shed fifty-five pounds in eleven weeks and had a silicone band fitted in his stomach. If it had not been for his check trousers, lurid even on a man famous for his lack of fashion sense, he would have looked positively athletic.

Another season, another attempt to get his life back on track and, in all likelihood, another disappointment. But so long as John Daly was prepared to risk that disappointment, his fans were not going to desert him. They, too, were in for the long haul.

Perhaps what was most remarkable about John Daly selling T-shirts at the 2009 Masters was not that he had the nerve to do it, but the warmth of the welcome he received from golf fans, who flocked to buy his wares, be photographed with him, get his signature. It would be too much to call Daly 'the people's champion', but he has probably attracted more love – not admiration – than many of his more illustrious contemporaries, Tiger Woods included.

That may not be fair, or rational. It is not an assertion that can be supported by the kind of statistics found in golf magazines. But when you see Daly on the golf course, with his ragbag army of supporters, as badly dressed as him, willing him to do well, the truth of it can hardly be disputed.

Professional golfers as a breed are a pretty bland lot: decent, hard-working, immaculately turned out, scrupulously honest on the course; but without the emotional turbulence of their counterparts in other sports. They do not make you worship them and despair of them at the same time – the way George Best did in football.

Daly, like Best, has tapped into the innate generosity in human nature, our willingness to forgive almost anything if certain preconditions are met. An alcoholic with a kind heart – and Daly has done far more than his share of charity work – will always trump a teetotaller with a less kind heart.

As a sportsman, in the Corinthian sense, Daly has never made the grade. The moments when he has lost the plot – taken a quadruple bogey, then stopped trying for the rest of the round – have revealed an unattractive lack of courtesy towards his playing companions. No wonder, despite his two majors, he has never represented America in the Ryder Cup. He lacks the humility of a team-player: he is too absorbed with fighting his own demons.

But if fans are drawn to him, it is not simply because he is an exciting golfer, hitting the ball unfeasible distances with his let-it-rip swing: it is also because he embodies virtues that transcend his shortcomings. Resilience. Determination. Dignity in the midst of indignity. Even at his lowest ebb, he has been capable of kindness, even sweetness.

'I'll tell you what real courage is,' wrote Harper Lee in *To Kill a Mockingbird*. 'It's not a man with a gun in his hand.

It's when you know you're licked before you begin, but you see it through anyway, no matter what. You rarely win, but sometimes you do.'

When the conversation at the nineteenth hole turns to John Daly, the refrain is always the same. 'What a waste!' The American won two majors before he was thirty, which very few other players have achieved. He promised so much, and threw it all away. If only he had looked after himself better . . .

But once that conversation is over, the other John Daly – the one who was not a quitter, but a survivor, coming back time after time, even if only to endure more humiliation, more disappointment – comes gradually into focus. He has made so many bad choices in his life that even his admirers lost count. But he has never lost his appetite for making one last despairing effort.

Suzanne Lenglen: Daring to Bare

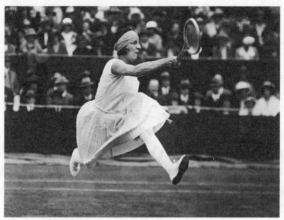

For such a widely admired quality, courage is oddly elastic. As the context changes, so does the nature of courage. The playing field is not level. Something that might have been daring in 1954 would have been run-of-the-mill by 1964, when everyone was doing it. A course of action that might be highly courageous in Mr A calls for no courage at all from Ms B – it is second nature to her.

If the athlete Hassiba Boulmerka had been raised in Italy, not Algeria, her sporting journey would have been relatively simple. Her talents as a runner – she won gold in the 1500m at the Barcelona Olympics – would have brought her fame and fortune. There would have been no downside to her success, no boos mingled with the applause. But growing up in a Muslim country, at a time when Islamic fundamentalism was on the rise, Boulmerka had to run the gauntlet of disapproval. It was as if a hurdle had been put in her lane.

A woman in running shorts was exposing so much more flesh than was culturally acceptable that, far from being honoured for her success, Boulmerka became a virtual pariah. In the rural mosques, as her career took off, she was denounced as 'scandalous . . . running with bare legs in front of thousands of men . . . not worthy of a Muslim woman . . .'

The athlete fought her corner like a tigress. 'It was my upbringing to be rebellious,' she declared. 'You try to be your own person, not to fall into a particular category.' But the forces of conservatism were too strong for her. She was forced out of Algeria and had to do her training in Europe.

The taboos that Boulmerka broke, and the courage she needed to challenge them, recalled the taboo-breaking exploits of another great sporting pioneer: the incomparable, the outrageous Suzanne Lenglen.

In 2011 it is so hard to relate to the social attitudes of the 1920s that there is a danger of underestimating what Suzanne Lenglen did, and the bottle she needed to do it. Her achievements as a tennis player speak for themselves. The Frenchwoman won Wimbledon six times, the French Open six times, and was beaten only once during her entire career – when she retired in the middle of a match suffering from whooping cough. But her achievements as a woman – using sport as a stage on which to express herself – were even more remarkable.

Lenglen died young, succumbing to anaemia when she was just thirty-nine, but she left an indelible mark on the history of her times. The world after Suzanne Lenglen was

very different from the world before Suzanne Lenglen –
not least because of social changes that she had helped to
bring about.

When she won the first of her Wimbledon titles, in
1919, her opponent, Lambert Chambers, the dominant
player of the Edwardian era, was wearing a corset, petticoats, white stockings, a full-sleeved white blouse and a
skirt that covered her ankles. That was what women tennis
players wore, as they always had. It was a uniform, theoret-
ically variable, but only at the cost of being conspicuous,
standing out from the crowd. It may not have been comfortable, but then neither, when you think about it, are the
business suits and ties that millions of men still wear – and
will go on wearing until someone sufficiently prominent
dares to be different. The herd instinct can be brutally
inflexible.

Enter, sans corset, sans petticoats, with bare arms, and a
skirt that exposed her calves, the twenty-year-old Suzanne
Lenglen, a tennis-playing prodigy from France. The
Wimbledon faithful were speechless. Good God, when she
ran across the court, or rose to hit a volley, you could even
see her thighs! On the manicured lawns of SW19, before
the stern gaze of Queen Mary, that unreconstructed
Victorian, a revolution was taking place.

Lenglen had not only reinterpreted the existing dress
code, tweaked it here and there. She had torn it up and
introduced a whole new one of her own. She was not clas-
sically good-looking, but what she had she flaunted, and
how.

The next year Lenglen was back at Wimbledon in a
tight-fitting blouse and an even shorter skirt, made of white
silk. Her jaunty bandeaus made her instantly recognisable –
spectators struck bets on what colour bandeau she would be

wearing for a given match. She wore full make-up on court, and would touch it up between games, when she also liked to take a swig of brandy. After the match, she would sweep from the court in a full-length fur coat. In a loser, her antics would have made her look ridiculous. In a winner, a champion who carried all before her, they were glorious, an exhilarating antidote to the drabness of the times.

Like radicals in other walks of life, Lenglen paid a price for swimming against the tide. To many, she was not a champion of her sex, but a traitor to it. Her costumes, sneered the American tennis player Bill Tilden, made her look like 'a cross between a primadonna and a streetwalker'. Off court, her many lovers, some married, made her an object of scandal and derision.

When Lenglen turned professional, outraging the tennis establishment, with its strict amateurism, she raised another storm. It took guts, like many of the things she did in her life. 'Only wealthy persons are able to compete at Wimbledon,' she said, with fine indignation. 'Is that fair? Does it advance the sport? Does it make tennis more popular? Or does it tend to suppress and hinder an enormous amount of tennis talent lying dormant in the bodies of young men and women whose names are not in the social register?' Stirring sentiments – but, in the class-conscious 1920s, the kind of sentiments that made more enemies than friends.

But then that was Lenglen all over. She could be her own worst enemy. She had a self-destructive streak. To the adoring French press, she was simply *La Divine*, a goddess. But her feet of clay captured the public imagination almost as much as her genius as a player.

The great paradox of Suzanne Lenglen is that a woman who was years ahead of her time, a pioneer with courage, was entirely devoid of the kind of natural feistiness her story implies. Far from being outgoing and self-confident, she had an emotional brittleness, allied to a strongly depressive streak, that distressed everyone who knew her.

Sickly as a child, then over-dependent on her father, who acted as her coach and mentor, she was prone to disintegrate at times of stress, weeping openly on court in a way that alienated many of her fans. She was like one of those nervous operatic divas who cancel at the first ticklings of a cough.

Her final Wimbledon, in 1926, should have been a personal triumph: she was a racing certainty to win the title for a record-equalling seventh time. But it turned into one of the saddest fiascos in the history of the Championships.

In one of her early matches, Lenglen unwittingly kept Queen Mary waiting for half an hour – there had been a misunderstanding about when the match was due on court. There were a few boos from the crowd – nothing a stronger woman could not have handled – but when Lenglen realised what had happened, she fell down in a faint. The player later withdrew from the tournament altogether and, despite efforts to make her change her mind, would never play at Wimbledon again.

It was an unworthy finale to a magnificent career. Whatever happened to the dashing twenty-year-old of seven years before, the bare-legged revolutionary, galvanising her sport with her groundbreaking approach to fashion?

Lenglen was a genius, a one-off, one of the great originals. And if it seems an exaggeration to credit her with courage, just remember what happened to her contemporary, the American swimmer Ethelda Bleibtrey, who won three gold medals at the 1920 Olympics in Antwerp.

In 1919, the same year that Lenglen made her debut at

Wimbledon, Bleibtrey was arrested at a public swimming-pool in the States and charged with 'nude swimming'. What had she done? Gone skinny-dipping? Nothing of the kind. She had simply removed her stockings at a pool where it was forbidden to 'bare the lower female extremities for public bathing'. In 1919 respectable women did not do these things.

Very few of the freedoms that women enjoy today were won without a struggle. They had to be fought for, tooth and nail – even on the manicured lawns of London SW19.

Jackie Robinson: The Guts Not to Fight Back

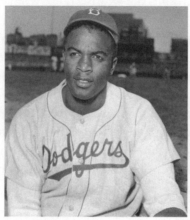

'A life is not important,' Jackie Robinson once said, 'except in the impact it has on other lives.'

His own short, revolutionary life was a textbook example.

Born in 1919, the year Suzanne Lenglen made her debut at Wimbledon, and dead of heart failure by his mid-fifties, Robinson enjoys a hallowed place in American sporting history, indeed in American history generally.

On 15 April 1947, a date known to every baseball fan, he became the first black player to appear in the Major League. Twenty-six thousand fans, more than half of them black, turned out at Ebbets Field to watch Robinson make his debut for the Brooklyn Dodgers. Not all of them were happy. And not all of them were relaxed. But they had come to see history made, and they were not disappointed.

The unthinkable had become thinkable. There would be no going back.

Sport, not for the first time, had sent a message that reverberated around the world.

Jackie Robinson was a towering figure, who made a huge impact, but one aspect of his career is worth underscoring: his steadfastness of purpose, often in the face of extreme provocation. As a young man, growing up in a world of bigotry, he was the reverse of steadfast: he was combustible, quick to take offence. But he had to learn to channel his anger, make it his servant, not his master. He had to learn to bite his tongue, bide his time. He had to suffer in silence – sometimes the most courageous course of all.

Born in Georgia, the son of a sharecropper, grandson of a slave, Robinson later moved to Pasadena, California, where his sporting ability soon became apparent. A career in baseball beckoned, playing in one of the Negro Leagues dotted around the country – the sport was still racially segregated, thanks to a long-standing gentlemen's agreement known as the 'baseball colour line'. Yet after the attack on Pearl Harbor in 1941, sport had to take a back seat. Robinson was drafted into the US Army and wound up a second lieutenant, assigned to a unit based in Fort Hood in Texas. But he never saw active service.

A celebrated incident on a bus – the driver told Robinson to move to the back of the bus, but he refused – led to him being court-martialled. In the eyes of some of the white officers in his unit, he was 'an uppity black man' who needed to be taken down a peg or two. The charges were dismissed, and Robinson received an honourable discharge, but he had learned an important lesson: if you wanted to bring about a change in attitudes, you had to be prepared to fight your corner.

In 1945, the first baseball season after the war, Robinson played for the Kansas City Monarchs, a Negro League team. He had little choice. It was not a happy experience: on a salary of $400 a month, playing in run-down stadiums, he felt underpaid, undervalued. When Branch Rickey, the president of the Brooklyn Dodgers, approached him with an alternative offer, he was ripe for the plucking.

Rickey was no anti-racist liberal, in the modern sense, but a hard-headed businessman. He could see that the days of the Negro Leagues were numbered, and wanted to be in a position to take advantage of desegregation when it finally reached his beloved baseball.

He proposed that Robinson play the 1946 season in the Montreal Royals, a minor-league 'farm team' for future Dodgers players. If he did well for the Royals, and coped with the racial abuse likely to come his way, he would get his chance for the Dodgers the following season. Rickey did not want a young hothead, however talented, who might start a brawl: he wanted someone who, in the words of the Good Book, could turn the other cheek.

The exchange between the two men on the subject of cheek-turning has entered baseball folklore.

Rickey: I know you're a good ballplayer. What I don't know is whether you have the guts.

Robinson: Mr Rickey, are you looking for a Negro who is afraid to fight back?

Rickey: No, Robinson. I'm looking for a ballplayer with guts enough not to fight back.

The deal was sealed, the two men shook hands on it, and on 23 October 1945, Rickey announced to a still sceptical world that Robinson had signed for the Montreal Royals, affiliated to the Dodgers. The Noble Experiment – as it was quickly hailed – had begun.

For Robinson, it was a baptism of fire. In Montreal itself, he quickly won over the fans, becoming the star performer in the side. But when the Royals were on the road, often staying in segregated hotels, the story changed. Their spring training schedule in Florida was continually disrupted. Some ballparks refused to host games involving Robinson; at another game, the police chief threatened to stop the game if he did not leave the field. A traditional Southern exhibition tour had to be cancelled altogether. Montreal might be ready for a black baseball player. Whole swathes of America were not.

His debut for the Dodgers the following season took place against a background of hostility. Even some of his team-mates were unsupportive. With mutiny brewing, manager Leo Durocher had to tell his team: 'I don't care if the guy is yellow or black, or if he has stripes like a fuckin' zebra. I'm the manager of this team and I say he plays.' Splendid sentiments – though what Durocher said next, in its way, is just as revealing: 'What's more, I say he can make us all rich.' The Dodgers dressing-room was not suddenly filled with liberals. Expressions of high moral principle had to be sugared with appeals to naked self-interest.

There came rumblings of resentment from other Major League teams, despite public expressions of support for Robinson. The St Louis Cardinals threatened to go on strike if Robinson played and rescinded the threat only when told they would be suspended from the league if they did not.

In a match against the Philadelphia Phillies, a week after Robinson made his debut, opposing players openly called him a 'nigger' from their dugout and yelled that he should 'go back to the cotton fields'. From the stands, match after match, came a steady stream of abuse. There was sulphur in the air.

If Robinson had to show extraordinary self-restraint, some of his fellow players also deserve credit. Pee Wee Reese, a Brooklyn team-mate, in an iconic gesture, put his arm around Robinson in sympathy after he had attracted a volley of racial abuse from fans in Cincinnati. 'You can hate a man for many reasons,' Reese said. 'Colour is not one of them.' Hank Greenberg, the veteran Jewish player, who had had to endure a mountain of prejudice himself, advised Robinson to let his baseball do the talking and beat the racists on the field.

Robinson did just that, helping the Dodgers to the 1947 World Series, which they lost to the New York Yankees. It was the first World Series to be televised, which was also significant. The lessons of the ballpark could now reach a wider audience. The tide was turning.

In a very few years, the Noble Experiment could be deemed an unqualified success. A black baseball player in the Major League ceased to be controversial. The abuse from the stands died down. Segregated hotels and restaurants began to change their policies. The way had been paved for the civil rights movement of the 1960s. Where baseball had led, society would follow.

But we should not forget the courage needed by one lonely figure when the experiment was in its infancy.

'I know that I must still prepare my children to meet obstacles and prejudices,' Robinson wrote in 1952:

But I can tell them, too, that they will never face
some of these prejudices because other people have
gone before them . . . Many of today's dogmas will
have vanished by the time they grow into adults . . .
There is nothing static in free people. There is no
Middle Ages logic so strong that it can stop the
human tide flowing forward. I do not believe that
every person, in every walk of life, can succeed in
spite of any handicap. That would be perfection. But
I do believe that what I was able to attain came to be
because we put behind the dogmas of the past to
discover the truth of today, and perhaps the greatness
of tomorrow.

Under the spotlight of sport, Jackie Robinson had borne
brave witness to his simple heartfelt credo: 'I believe in the
human race. I believe in the warm heart. I believe in man's
integrity. I believe in the goodness of a free society. And I
believe that society can remain good only as long as we are
willing to fight for it.'

What a man. When they made a movie of his life, only
one person had the charisma to play the main character.

Jackie Robinson himself.

Eric Liddell: The Flying Scotsman

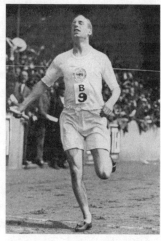

GETTY IMAGES

Jackie Robinson may have had to swim against a raging tide, but he had history with him, and he knew it. To swim against the tide when history is not on your side takes, arguably, even greater courage.

In 2011 the refusal of Eric Liddell to run on a Sunday at the 1924 Olympics – immortalised in the film *Chariots of Fire* – seems honourable, but quixotic. The principles the Scot fought for have been overtaken by events. Millions of Christians happily play sport every Sunday of the year; no professional sportsman could survive at the top level if he was not prepared to do the same. Liddell, the son of missionaries, and later a missionary himself, seems like a relic from a bygone era, a dinosaur. But his courage, his adamantine resolve, must be saluted. In the shifting sands of sport, he was a rock.

'God made me fast,' Liddell once said. 'And when I run, I feel His pleasure.' If he said that today, he would be laughed at. If he said it fifty years from now, he would probably be treated for schizophrenia. But he believed it, and if ever a man stuck to his beliefs, it was Eric Liddell. Probably no athlete in Olympic history so epitomised a truth of universal relevance, whether you are a Christian or not: there are more important things than winning medals.

Far too much of the history of sport is written by the winners, or about the winners – to the point where success is overvalued and other sporting virtues eclipsed. We need the odd Eric Liddell, a renouncer of glory, a loser by deliberate choice, to keep us on our feet.

Born in China, educated in Edinburgh, Liddell was the outstanding all-round athlete of his generation, representing his country at rugby as well as being a superlative sprinter, admiringly nicknamed 'The Flying Scotsman'. In the spring of 1924 he broke the British 100-yards record in a time that would stand for more than thirty years. Success in the 100m at the Paris Olympics, held later that year, would have been a formality, if the organisers had not scheduled the final for a Sunday. Liddell, who never ran on the Sabbath, was out of the race before the starting-gun had been fired.

In the movie, the Scot finds out that the 100m final has been scheduled for a Sunday only as he is boarding the cross-Channel ferry en route to Paris. Cue much anguished soul-searching, with the Prince of Wales and others trying to persuade him to change his mind. Good cinema, bad history. Liddell had known about the scheduling for months, realised that he would not be able to win the 100m gold, and redirected his energies to training for the 400m final.

But even before the artistic licence, it was a great sporting story, with an admirable, if rather dour hero. Liddell was not alone among his contemporaries in the attitude he took to the Sabbath. The great England cricketer Jack Hobbs quietly insisted that he would not play on a Sunday. On a tour of India, after his position became known, a one-day match scheduled for a Sunday was discreetly rearranged. Dorothy Round, the 1934 Wimbledon Ladies' Singles Champion, was equally uncompromising. 'I will never consent to play tennis on a Sunday.' But Liddell's stance has become the most celebrated, not simply because of the movie, but because it was so costly to his medal prospects.

Out of contention in the 100m because of the scheduling, no one fancied Liddell for a medal in the 400m. It was not his distance. But in one of the best Olympic twists, the Scot was not going to let a little detail like that get in his way.

Just before the race – and this bit was not invented for the cinema, it was one of those stranger-than-fiction moments – an American masseur thrust a piece of paper into his hand, with a quotation from 1 Samuel: 'Those who honour me, I will honour.' It acted like a last-minute injection of steroids. Liddell not only won the race, still clutching the piece of paper, but smashed the world record. He had secured his legacy.

After retiring from athletics, Liddell threw himself into a new life as a missionary in China. It was gruelling work, particularly after the outbreak of war and the Japanese invasion. There were still odd glimpses of the great athlete:

Liddell's daughter remembers her father sprinting to catch a wild hare when wartime rationing forced people to take desperate measures. But Olympic gold must have seemed a distant memory.

In 1943 Liddell was placed in an internment camp in Weifang (where he died of a brain tumour in February 1945). His fellow internees revered him as a model of Christian charity and compassion. He bore the appalling camp conditions with characteristic forbearance, and is now almost as fondly remembered in China as in Scotland. In the record-books, because he was born in China, he is even listed as China's first Olympic champion.

In 1991, as a result of an initiative by Edinburgh University, a memorial headstone was erected at the former internment camp in Weifang. It is inscribed with words from the Book of Isaiah that Eric Liddell used to quote in his sermons: 'They shall mount up with wings, as eagles; they shall run and not be weary.'

To those who erected the simple memorial, Liddell must have seemed a distant figure, wreathed in the mists of time: a sportsman whose very personal journey of faith would never be repeated. But, by an irony that the Scot would have savoured, his example had not been forgotten.

That very same year, 1991, the New Zealand rugby player Michael Jones had to wrestle with an identical crisis of conscience. A committed Christian, Jones refused to play on a Sunday, whether his country needed him or not. In 1987, when New Zealand won the World Cup, he played in the quarter-final, missed out on the semi-final because it was played on a Sunday, but was then recalled for the final. But if fans respected his stance, it did not meet with universal approval. Even in God-fearing New Zealand, there is only one true religion – rugby.

The 1991 World Cup schedule meant that Jones would have to miss three matches if New Zealand were to defend their title successfully. When they fell short, losing in the semi-final to Australia – in a Sunday match played without Jones – the absent flanker took some of the criticism. Couldn't he just have bent his principles a teeny bit? This was the All Blacks versus the Wallabies. His intransigence on the issue later led to him being left out of the 1995 World Cup altogether.

A winner's medal sacrificed on the altar of principle . . . It was as if Eric Liddell had come back to life. Not all Christian sportsmen are good advertisements for their faith. Some are the very opposite. But Michael Jones wore his conscience lightly. The player nicknamed 'The Ice Man', for his coolness under pressure, was able to laugh at himself. Asked once how such a devout Christian could be such a ferocious tackler, he wryly replied: 'It is better to give than to receive.'

Conformity is the death of sport, and it will be a sad day, for all kinds of reasons, if every sportsman, without exception, feels obligated to give sport precedence over religious observation or family responsibilities.

The Flying Scotsman has an unassailable place among the sportsmen who dared to be different despite what anyone thought of them.

Alex Ferguson: A Manager Earns His Corn

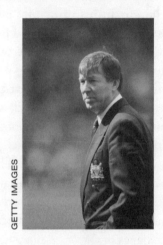

GETTY IMAGES

How to break the bad news?

In the world beyond sport, it can be the most agonising decision of all. You have to tell someone you love something that you know will hurt them, perhaps damage your relationship irreparably. Do you just come straight out with it? Or do you dither? Spend sleepless nights worrying? Rehearse what you are going to say, then tear up that speech and start a new one? Wimp out and write a letter? Break out in a sweat at the thought of the moment when you have to stop the shilly-shallying and look the other person in the eye?

I know what I do. And I suspect 99 per cent of the population would give the same answer.

Which is why I have always admired the courage that

Alex Ferguson displayed one May evening in 1990. It was a private moment. There were no cameras present. In that sense, it is different in nature from the other episodes in this book, which were played out on a public stage. But did the protagonist of the drama need to show guts, nerve, strength of character? Beyond question. In fact, it is one of the defining moments in one of the most illustrious careers in sport.

Lovers of sporting what-ifs always dwell on the third-round FA Cup tie between Nottingham Forest and Manchester United in January 1990. United sneaked through 1-0, won the European Cup Winners' Cup the following year, and have never looked back. But what if they had lost at Forest? Would Ferguson have kept his job? We will never know. It is one of the great imponderables.

But that third-round tie was only part of the story in 1990. If the Forest match was, in Ferguson's famous phrase, squeaky bum time, the pressure on the Scot was just as intense in the later stages of the competition. United won a nervy semi-final against Oldham Athletic, but only after a replay, having drawn the first match 3-3. When the Wembley final, against Crystal Palace, followed an identical script, with the two sides deadlocked at 3-3 after extra time, the manager could have been forgiven for tearing his hair out in clumps and hitting the bottle in the wee small hours.

Instead, before the replay, Ferguson took one of the coolest, bravest decisions of his entire managerial career. He dropped one of his favourite sons, a player he had brought with him to Old Trafford from Aberdeen, a fellow Scot, a friend – goalkeeper Jim Leighton.

How easy the decision looks now, with the hindsight of history. When a team is leaking goals, drawing games 3-3, the goalkeeper is bound to come under scrutiny. Against Crystal Palace in the first match, Leighton had been nervous, flapping at crosses, making handling errors. His confidence appeared shot. Les Sealey, the man Ferguson brought in to replace him, kept a clean sheet in the replay, which is all that can be asked of any goalkeeper. Perhaps Leighton would have kept a clean sheet too. Academic. The dropping of Leighton worked. QED. It was a managerial masterstroke.

But, at the time, dropping Leighton was a long, long way from being an obvious solution. There was real agony in the decision, both for the discarded goalkeeper and for the manager who had to break the news to him. In Ferguson's autobiography, *Managing My Life*, when he describes the moment he took Leighton aside the day before the match, his understated choice of words howls out the emotional enormity of what took place. 'He took it very badly. I felt so sorry for him.'

What did the two men say to each other? One can try to fill in the dialogue but, in a sense, the scene does not need dialogue: it is starkly simple. In the space of a few momentous minutes, two men who had shared so much, been blood brothers in the glory days at Aberdeen, had fallen out for all eternity.

Deep in his heart, like the hero of a Greek tragedy who foresees his destiny, Ferguson must have known what would happen when he dropped Leighton. He knew, before he had said a word, that the goalkeeper would be inconsolable. That was the genuine pathos of the situation.

Archie Knox, his second-in-command since his Aberdeen days, had urged him not to do it: he knew both men, all too well. But Ferguson had to wield the axe. It was, as he saw it, his professional duty. His destiny.

'It was animal instinct,' he was quoted as saying in the *Sun*. 'I smelled danger after the first Wembley game. I knew Jim had to be dropped.'

Alex Ferguson is such a compelling figure that there can hardly be a football fan in the country who would not like to be a fly on the wall at one of his half-time team talks, when he is laying into his players, giving them the famous hair-dryer treatment. But who would want to have been a fly on the wall when Ferguson told poor Jim Leighton he was dropping him? It must have been an excruciating conversation, leaving wounds that have never healed.

Professional sport can be very cruel.

The aftermath is almost as painful to read about as the dropping of Leighton itself. The goalkeeper basically fell into a sulk from which he took years to emerge.

After United had won the replay and Bryan Robson had lifted the FA Cup, the team met up with their wives and families at Wembley Station. Ferguson wrote in his autobiography that he tried to have a word with Leighton's wife, Linda, but she gave him a V-sign and turned her back on him. 'That stung,' admitted Ferguson.

Even though United had won the Cup, some of the next day's papers accused the manager of having betrayed the goalkeeper who had served him so loyally for so long. 'That allegation has hung in the air over the years,' writes Ferguson, 'and in a way Leighton has been glorified.'

His rebuttal is typically trenchant: 'To put it bluntly, I believe Jim was selfish . . . I profoundly regret that our relationship deteriorated, but I have no remorse.' And what fair-minded neutral would not take his side? What is a manager paid for if not to take tough decisions? How can any football club prosper if the manager is not free to choose the team he wants for each match, the team he thinks will best serve the needs of the club?

Later that summer, when Leighton was playing for

Scotland in the World Cup in Italy, and had made a fatal blunder in a match against Brazil, Ferguson rang to commiserate, but was rebuffed. The next season, with Les Sealey now the first-choice goalkeeper at Old Trafford, Leighton was sent on loan to Sheffield United and Arsenal, before being sold to Dundee. He was never quite the same goalkeeper again, although he recovered his form sufficiently to be picked for Scotland in the 1998 World Cup in France, just short of his fortieth birthday.

The sad thing is that, although it is Alex Ferguson's courage that shines through this episode, the goalkeeper he dropped was also renowned for his bravery. 'His grit and courage were never in question,' said Ferguson, after Leighton performed heroics for Aberdeen against Celtic in a Scottish Cup final, playing with stitches in his hand after he had nearly severed his fingers using an electric lawnmower. If the roll of the dice had been different, he could have been remembered for that bravery, a Scottish Bert Trautmann.

Instead, as the world knows, it all ended in tears.

Football. Bloody hell.

Dean Jones: 'Get Me a Real Australian'

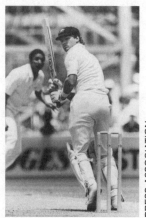

'I played a bad shot and got out,' said Dean Jones of the most infamous moment of his career. During the 2006 series between Sri Lanka and South Africa, he was commentating for Ten Sports, the Australian broadcaster, when a catch fell to Hashim Amla, the bearded South African player, a devout Muslim. 'The terrorist has got another wicket,' quipped Jones, thinking he was off air. When a microphone picked up the comment, he was out of his job within hours, sunk in a storm of protest.

'It was a silly and completely insensitive thing to say,' Jones acknowledged, 'and obviously it was never supposed to be heard over the air. I am truly sorry to have caused offence to anybody.' He was quick to apologise to Amla. Ironically, his faux pas came at a time when his reputation had never been higher. Just weeks before, he had been made a Member of the Order of Australia for services to charity fundraising.

Only those with long memories remembered Jones's finest hour as a cricketer: one of the gutsiest, most heroic innings ever played, a sporting epic, with a big-hearted young hero, and a white-knuckle ambulance ride worthy of a Hollywood blockbuster.

The innings happened towards the start of his career, when Jones, who played for Victoria, was trying to cement a place in the national team under the captaincy of Allan Border. The mid-1980s were a transitional time for Australian cricket. The team of Dennis Lillee, Rodney Marsh and the Chappell brothers had broken up, and replacements of their calibre had not yet been found. If ever there was a moment for a plucky young batsman to take centre stage . . .

Jones had played only two Tests before being selected to tour India in 1986, but was now offered the all-important number-three position in the batting order, the one forever associated with Don Bradman. 'Don't force things,' Border told him. 'Just play your natural game.'

It was a tough challenge – the cricketing graveyard is not short of players who have been told to play their natural game – but when Jones came out to bat in the first Test in Madras, modern Chennai, he made a confident start. By close of play on the first day, he had reached 56 not out, and Australia were in command of the match, thanks to a hundred by David Boon. On a searingly hot day – humidity topped eighty degrees – Jones had enjoyed himself too much to notice the weather. He went to bed exhausted but happy.

His problems started the next morning, after he had

reached his century. He was dehydrated and cramping badly. And the longer he batted, the more dehydrated he got. Using his feet against the spinners was impossible. Even running a single became difficult.

'By the time I got to 130, I was starting to vomit,' Jones remembers. 'I had pins and needles all over my body. I couldn't bend to sweep and could hardly move my legs. Then I started to urinate involuntarily. My body was going haywire and entering into shock. I was completely out of it.'

Sanity demanded that Jones retire hurt, then resume his innings later. But sanity never got a look in. With the help of regular ministrations from the team physio, Errol Alcott, the Australian soldiered grimly on. The Indian fielders could see how sick he was, and offered him bottles of sweet lime soda to drink, but Jones just vomited it straight back up.

'I lost seven kilos in the heat, but I needed to do it. I had to put myself through the wall to get where I needed to be. This was my Mount Everest. I had to climb it to prove to myself that I could compete at this level. But by gee, it was bloody hard work.'

When Jones got to 170, common sense finally prevailed, and he told Allan Border, who was batting at the other end, that he could not go on. 'Then I'll get a real Australian instead,' his captain said. 'We need a tough Queenslander out here' – a reference to Greg Ritchie, the next man in. The ploy worked. Jones gritted his teeth and carried on.

By tea, he had reached 202, and had to be dragged physically into the shower by team-mates – he could hardly put two steps together on his own. Then they padded him up again and pushed him back on to the field – minus his box and thigh-pad in the chaos. By now, as far as Jones was concerned, everything was just a blur. He was out shortly after tea for 210 and, in obvious distress, had to be rushed to hospital in an ambulance.

Even now, the drama was not over. Five Indian doctors, excited at the prospect of being able to treat an Australian cricketer, fought over Jones in the back of the ambulance. The driver, convinced that the Australian had suffered a heart attack, careered through the narrow streets of Madras, taking the bends so fast that Jones kept falling off his bed, sending more muscles into spasm. Pleas to slow down were ignored. More vomiting. More groans of pain. A simple sporting injury had spiralled comically out of control.

And all because a pig-headed young Australian was too proud to retire hurt.

Dean Jones's heroics alone would have been enough to make the 1986 Madras Test a famous sporting encounter. But, on this occasion, the scriptwriter was working over-time. A dramatic match ended in a tie, only the second in Test history. It also marked a turning point in Australian fortunes. After a few years in the doldrums, the team was on the march again.

A year later, Australia won the World Cup in India. Two years after that, they regained the Ashes during the 1989 tour in England. Jones, now a fixture in the side, played a starring role on both occasions. By the time he played his last Test, in 1992, Australia were set on the path to world domination – thanks not least to Jones himself and the unquenchable spirit he had shown in Madras. His innings was more than a personal triumph: it was a watershed.

Would things have turned out differently if Jones had done the sensible thing, retired hurt and sought proper treatment instead of driving his body to the brink of col-lapse? Who can say? In our hunger for sporting heroes, it is easy to exaggerate a feel-good story, or wrench it out of context. It was only a cricket match, albeit a particularly exciting one. But one aspect of what happened at Madras is surely worth remarking.

In sport as in life, time never stands still. The tide turns. The momentum shifts from one side to another. As England cricket fans of a certain age will remember, the Australian sides of the early and mid-1980s were regularly out-Beefed by the England of the Botham era. They had some fine individuals but, as a unit, lacked grit, resolve, mental toughness. They seemed diffident, unsure of themselves, almost as if they were afraid to win. When Kim Hughes tearfully quit the captaincy in 1984, it seemed symptomatic of a deeper malaise.

After Madras, there was no such diffidence. And there has been no trace of it ever since. One mad, mulish individual, in so much pain he could hardly hold a cricket bat, saw to that.

Alice Marble: The Letter That Changed Tennis

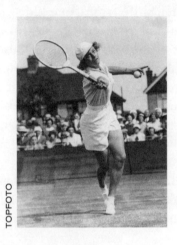

TOPFOTO

On a Beaufort scale of courage, how do you begin to know where to put Alice Marble?

In an amazing, incident-packed life, the former Wimbledon champion had to dare so much, endure so much, overcome so much, that she is several sporting heroines wrapped into one.

On court, she was ahead of her time, a pioneer: the first woman to base her game on serve-and-volley tactics, and the first to wear shorts on court. Like Suzanne Lenglen, she dared to be different, to challenge the conventional view of how a sportswoman should conduct herself in public. But her life off court revealed her real character. Her splendidly apt surname gives the merest hint of her emotional resilience.

Born in California in 1913, Marble lost her father in a car accident when she was seven, and had a tomboy childhood, hanging around ballparks with her brothers, matching them slug for slug at baseball. 'I won't play that sissy game!' she yelled, when they suggested that she take up some more ladylike sport. She quickly excelled at tennis, winning championships as a junior before rising to national prominence. Yet there were obstacles in her way. There always were with Alice Marble.

At fifteen, she was raped by a stranger at her local tennis club. The man was never caught or even identified. At twenty-one, after collapsing before a match in Paris, she was diagnosed with tuberculosis, spent long months in a sanatorium, and was told she would never play tennis again. Instead of bowing to the inevitable, she simply checked out of the sanatorium and sought a second opinion. Not tuberculosis, said the second doctor, just a severe case of pleurisy. Game on.

By the late 1930s, Marble had established herself as the leading player of her generation, winning Wimbledon in 1939. At the post-tournament ball, her partner was the men's champion, Bobby Riggs, who would later tangle with Billie Jean King in the Battle of the Sexes.

When war intervened, Marble was at the peak of her career. Hitler robbed her of the procession of Grand Slam titles that would have cemented her place among the all-time greats. Not that tennis was uppermost in her thoughts. After a whirlwind romance, she married an Air Force pilot, got pregnant, then miscarried after a car accident. Days later, her husband was killed in action after his plane was shot down over Germany. Marble, at her lowest ebb, tried to commit suicide. Even the doughtiest fighters are prey to moments of despair. But she quickly recovered her zest for life.

The next chapter in her life is the murkiest, much of the detail still veiled in secrecy. US Intelligence recruited the widowed, now professional tennis star as a spy. Her mission was to make contact with a former lover, resident in Switzerland, and use him to get vital financial information about the Nazis. It all went badly wrong. Marble was shot and wounded, before being rescued and flown back to the States.

For a time, appropriately, the tennis-champion-turned-spy edited the comic-strip magazine *Wonder Woman*. Versatile and indefatigable, limitlessly resourceful, she was a multi-tasker before the term had been invented. Marble even enjoyed success as a football commentator on a New York radio station.

But, even now that she had retired from top-flight tennis, her work was not done. One of the bravest actions of her whole career lay in the future.

In July 1950, Alice Marble wrote a letter.

It was an open letter, published in the *American Lawn Tennis Magazine*, and it now seems charmingly old-fashioned, both in its language and its sentiments. In the genteel world of American tennis in 1950, it acted like a stick of dynamite. The author was not articulating some fashionable liberal consensus: she was challenging a highly illiberal one because she, Alice Marble, found it odious.

At issue was a simple question of principle. Should Althea Gibson, a black player, be allowed to compete at the US Open at Forest Hills? As things stood, even three years after Jackie Robinson had broken through the colour barrier in baseball, and black football players were starting to be seen in the NFL, tennis remained strictly segregated. Gibson and other black players were stuck in the ghetto of the American Tennis Association and debarred from Grand Slam events. Someone had to take up the cudgels on their behalf, and that someone was Alice Marble.

'Miss Gibson is over a very cunningly wrought barrel,' she wrote, 'and I can only hope to loosen a few of its staves with one lone opinion. But if tennis is a game for ladies and gentlemen, it is also time we acted a little bit more like gentle people and less like sanctimonious hypocrites . . . If Althea Gibson represents a challenge to the present crop of women players, it is only fair that they should meet that challenge on the courts.'

If Gibson were not given the opportunity to compete, Marble concluded, it would be 'an ineradicable mark against a game to which I have devoted most of my life, and I would be bitterly ashamed'.

Powerful words – and, to their credit, the sanctimonious chiefs at Forest Hills took heed. Within weeks, Gibson was competing in the US Open, before going on to Grand Slam glory, winning back-to-back Wimbledon titles in 1957 and 1958.

She was an outstanding player who, without Alice Marble's intervention, would probably have made it to the top anyway. But she would have had to wait longer before receiving her rightful due. It took two further years for a black male player, Reginald Weir, to play in the US Open; more than ten for a black golfer, Charlie Sifford, to be admitted to the PGA tour. Racial prejudice in sport did not melt away by itself. It had to be eradicated by men and women with the courage to stand up to it – while still heavily outnumbered, prophets without honour.

'No matter what accomplishments you make,' Althea Gibson once said, 'somebody helps you.' After Marble died, in 1990, she saluted her as 'a great, kind and gracious lady' and 'the one person that stood up for me in the tennis world'. She knew, better than anyone, the debt she owed her fellow champion.

In the bigoted world of 1950 America, nothing would have been easier than for Marble to say nothing for a few more years, and wait until the US Open was ready to welcome a black player with open arms. But Alice Marble was never one to shy away from a challenge. By taking an unequivocal stance, and through the force of her personality, she shamed the tennis world into doing the decent thing.

More than a decade before the civil rights movement of the 1960s, she saw the iniquity of racial segregation in tennis and denounced it with thrilling clarity.

The Ballad of Haydn Bunton

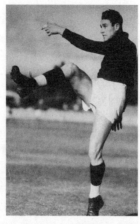

AFL PHOTOS

Twenty years before Alice Marble wrote her famous letter, on the other side of the world an iconic Australian sportsman exhibited the same courage, the same humanity, the same moral leadership.

If you want to get an Aussie sports fan to cry like a baby – normally a hard ask, not even worth attempting unless you have an onion to hand – just find a recording of 'The Ballad of Haydn Bunton', composed in 2003 by the folk singer Ken Mansell. It is a shamelessly sentimental piece, celebrating the man often described as the greatest of all Australian rules footballers.

Born in Albury, New South Wales, in 1911, Bunton was a contemporary of Don Bradman and, like the Don, lit up the Depression years with his feats on the sports field. As a young man, he played cricket with Bradman, and some judges reckoned Bunton the better player – a thought to give England cricket fans sleepless nights. But Bunton made his name in the Victorian Football League (VFL), the precursor of the modern Australian Football League.

He played for Fitzroy, a suburb of Melbourne, and, at that time, one of the stronger clubs in the VFL. Fitzroy the club no longer exists: it was forced to close in the 1990s, squeezed out by bigger clubs. But somehow the demise of the Roys only adds lustre to their glory days between the wars, one of those fondly remembered golden ages – imperishable, irretrievable. The club may be no more, but the ghosts of players like Wilfred 'Chicken' Smallhorn will hover in the Fitzroy air for a long time to come.

Haydn Bunton blotted his copybook right at the start of his career – a salient reminder that even golden ages are rarely perfect. Fitzroy were so desperate to sign him that they offered him a one-off payment of $222, which was illegal under VFL rules. The player missed the 1930 season as a result, and when he started playing for Fitzroy in 1931 was on a salary of just $2 a week. During the day, he worked at Foys, a department store in Melbourne, and would practise sidesteps by weaving his way through crowds of shoppers. Oh to have been a fly on the wall in the haberdashery department.

On the field, Bunton was an immediate success, winning the Brownlow Medal, the highest individual honour in the game, in his first season, then winning it again the following year. He was a superlative athlete and a dashing, romantic figure, a gift to the balladist, and Ken Mansell lays it on with a trowel, as a good balladist should.

In the gloomy, hungry Thirties,
When Fitzroy folk were low,

A touch of Bunton magic
Could set all hearts aglow . . .

But it is when Doug Nicholls appears that the ballad has
you reaching for your handkerchief.

When little Dougie Nicholls
Came down from the scrub,
Football was a white man's game –
At Carlton he was snubbed.

Just an Aborigine,
They would not let him in.
No one saw his blinding pace,
Just the colour of his skin . . .

Sir Douglas Nicholls, KCVO, OBE, sportsman, pastor,
governor of South Australia, was a great man in his own
right, one of the most revered of all indigenous Australians.
He was born in 1906, on the Cummeragunja mission in
New South Wales, and like other Aborigines of his day,
had a wretched education. When he was eight, he had to
watch as his elder sister was forcibly taken from her family
by the police and put in the chillingly named Cootamundra
Training School for Girls.

Nicholls left school at thirteen, barely able to read and
write, then worked with his uncle on a sheep station. When
he moved to Melbourne in the early 1920s, he had no
money and nowhere to stay, so he slept in boxes at Victoria
Market.

He was a tiny man, just five foot two, but lightning-fast
and with great sporting promise. Although no formal bar
against Aboriginal players existed in the VFL, there had only

ever been a handful of them, all of whom faced an uphill struggle. As recorded in the ballad, Nicholls did play for Carlton in the 1926 season, but his team-mates froze him out. The trainers reputedly refused to treat him because he had black skin. For several seasons, Nicholls was reduced to playing for Northcote, a minor-league side, and performing in a travelling boxing troupe to supplement his income.

When Fitzroy signed him for the 1932 season, the club was taking a calculated gamble. In terms of racial tolerance, the Roys had a better track record than other VFL clubs. In 1904 Joe Johnson had become the first indigenous Australian to play in the VFL. Then there had been Norm Byron, who turned out for the Roys in 1918, before becoming well known as a singer and songwriter, the uncrowned poet laureate of the club. Yet the presence of an indigenous player in a team was still guaranteed to raise hackles.

For many ordinary fans, white Australia was not just a demographic reality, with whites accounting for 98 per cent of the population, but an article of faith. In *The Bulletin*, one of the most respected papers of the day, the editorial page carried the legend 'Australia for the White Man'. A lot of furniture of the period – as Haydn Bunton would have seen in Foys department store – was stamped with the words 'Made with White Labour'.

Someone had to find a better way. That someone was Haydn Bunton.

When he came into the Fitzroy dressing-room at the start of the 1932 season, and saw his new team-mate, a mass of nerves, he simply went across to Doug Nicholls, put his bag down next to his and gave him a little squeeze, as if to say: everything is going to be all right.

And everything was all right. The little Aborigine winger became a fixture in the club for most of the 1930s, admired and respected by all. A simple gesture of friendship – 'an arm around the shoulder of the black boy near the door', in the words of the ballad – had given a lead, and ensured that the casual racism that Nicholls had encountered at Carlton would not be replicated at Fitzroy.

Two different football clubs, two different suburbs of Melbourne and, as far as Doug Nicholls was concerned, two quite different experiences – not because Carlton was run by the Ku Klux Klan and Fitzroy was a hotbed of liberalism, but because one man was big enough to do the decent thing.

In contrast to some of the *Boy's Own* heroics elsewhere in the book, the courage Haydn Bunton displayed was of the quiet, understated variety. But does that make it any less laudable? You can see why the story appealed to the balladist, with its simple, wholesome moral.

When Pastor Douglas Nicholls
Was meek and scared and shy,
He found a mate in Bunton,
A man before his time.

Bunton was more than a good mate to Nicholls – he was so far ahead of his time that, in some respects, his time has not yet come. Even in 2011 Aborigines occupy an uneasy place in Australian society, subject to prejudice and discrimination. For every Cathy Freeman – the runner whom the country took to its heart after she won gold at the Sydney Olympics – there is an Aboriginal sportsman or woman whose career suffers because of the colour of their skin. Racism is not limited to one country or to one generation. It is omnipresent, and has to be confronted again and again and again.

Haydn Bunton was colour-blind in the finest sense. Unlike Doug Nicholls, his Fitzroy team-mate, who lived well into his nineties and became a national treasure, the great footballer was not destined to enjoy the life of an elder statesman: he died in a car crash in 1955. But he left an indelible mark on his times, for reasons that went far beyond his prowess as a sportsman.

Malcolm Marshall: The One-Armed Bandit

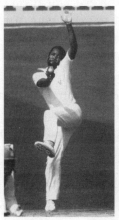

If Dean Jones came to epitomise the physical toughness of Australian cricket, the elusive X-factor that made them such formidable opponents, his counterpart in the West Indian team of the 1980s was the late, great Malcolm Marshall.

Marshall – 'Maco' to his friends – became one of the most fondly remembered cricketers ever to come out of the Caribbean. The Barbados-born fast bowler was forty-one when he died of cancer in 1999, but the tributes to him had an unstinting warmth that went beyond ritual expressions of regret. He was a genuinely nice, easy-going man, who had a touch of the old-fashioned Corinthian about him: someone who played the game for love, and did not take it over-seriously. Martin Crowe, the great

New Zealand batsman, summed the bowler up to perfection – 'furious but fair, and fantastic value in the bar'.

With his gold chains and flash suits, Marshall was as much showman as sportsman: one of those larger-than-life figures who command awe and affection in equal measure. He liked to win, but to win with panache, brio, rather than just grinding out results.

One of the best Marshall stories revolved around a match for Hampshire against Glamorgan in Pontypridd in the 1980s. At the start of the third day, Glamorgan had a slender second innings lead, but still had seven wickets in hand. Marshall, with swaggering assurance, phoned his golf club in Southampton from the dressing-room and booked a tee-time for four o'clock. He then took six of the remaining seven wickets himself, drove over a hundred miles and was on the tee by five past four, apologising to his playing companions for being late. It was like another episode from the golden age, when players puffed at Woodbines in the outfield and turned up in the dressing-room in their dinner jackets after a night on the tiles.

Another Marshall story features the Essex spin-bowlers, Ray East and David Acfield, celebrated pranksters on the county circuit. When he arrived at the ground, Marshall was surprised to see the two men, nervous tail-end rabbits, waiting to greet him. They even offered to carry his bag to the pavilion. 'Why?' asked the bemused fast bowler. 'Well, Mr Marshall,' came the answer, after much forelock-tugging, 'we thought you might consider a couple of half-volleys, and if they are nice and straight, we promise to miss them.'

In his prime for the West Indies, bowling alongside Joel Garner, Michael Holding and Colin Croft, Marshall struck terror into his opponents with his fast, skiddy action. Shorter than the other three, he was no less quick and no less hostile. Many regarded him as the greatest of them all: a bowler of relentless menace who could also bat a bit.

Fast bowlers are the ultimate sporting bullies, the ones who rule by fear. Many an opposing batsman was left battered and bruised after being on the receiving end of a Malcolm Marshall special. One of his victims, England opener Andy Lloyd, did not play for his country again after being hit on the helmet by a bouncer. But it could never be said of Marshall, as has been said of some fast bowlers, that he could give it out, but could not take it.

Not after what he did at Headingley in 1984.

In the folklore of cricket, the West Indies team that administered a famous 'blackwash' to England in 1984, then repeated the dose in the Caribbean two years later, ranks high among the greatest elevens of all time: the batting pyrotechnics of Greenidge, Haynes, Richards et al., backed by a fearsome battery of fast bowlers. But invincibility was not its birthright: it had to be earned.

It is easy to overlook the fact that the England team that succumbed 5-0 in 1984 had some formidable players of its own: Botham, Gower, Lamb and Willis, to name but four. At Lord's, in the second Test, England gave as good as they got for the first four days and only lost, after declaring, because of a double century of outrageous brilliance from Gordon Greenidge. At Headingley, in the next Test, again little separated the sides. England posted 270, thanks to a century by Allan Lamb, and West Indies in reply were 290 for nine, no more than a nose in front, when Malcolm Marshall decided to spice up the script.

In the England first innings, he had bowled just six overs, having hurt his hand fielding. He was taken to hospital, where X-rays showed that he had fractured his thumb in two places. He was not expected to bat, except in an emergency, and probably would not have batted at all if his team-mate Larry Gomes had not been closing in on a century. When the ninth West Indies wicket fell, the England players started making for the pavilion, and were surprised to see Marshall strolling to the crease, with a smile on his face and his left hand encased in plaster. Shades of Colin Cowdrey in 1963.

Unlike Cowdrey, who did not have to face a ball, Marshall was quickly into action, holding the bat with one hand to protect his broken thumb. With no point in defending, he chanced his one good arm. It was knockabout stuff and while Marshall enjoyed every minute, proceedings took on a carnival air. Mostly he swung and missed, although he did manage one four to third man, before being caught at slip by Ian Botham, after an entertaining cameo.

More importantly, Marshall had stayed around long enough to see Gomes through to his century. The West Indies had extended their first innings lead to 32. It was a slender advantage and, with one of their front-line bowlers out of action with a broken thumb . . .

What happened next is there in black and white in *Wisden*. Malcolm Marshall: 26 overs, 9 maidens, 53 runs, 7 wickets. Superb figures in any circumstances. Unimaginable in these.

The West Indies went on to win the match by eight wickets, and the series 5-0, and the *next* series against England 5-0. They bulldozed them, day after day, match after match. But would they have achieved such supremacy, demoralising the opposition, if a fast bowler with a broken thumb had not ignored the pain and produced the best bowling figures of his Test career?

For a spin bowler, an injury to the non-bowling arm would have been awkward, but no more than that. For Marshall, hurtling in to bowl, both arms pumping, every Headingley delivery must have been agony. He had to reduce his run to half its normal length. He had to fall back on his craft, his animal cunning, his reserves of determination.

The decisive breakthrough came in his second spell. At 104 for two, with David Gower and Graeme Fowler well set, England were doing nicely, more than seventy runs ahead with eight wickets in hand. Then Marshall got what he must have been dreading: a sharp return catch, jarring his bad thumb. He clung on to it, hopping up and down in pain, took another wicket almost immediately, then mopped up the tail. It was one of the legendary spells of bowling.

In the very next Test, by a strange quirk of fate, Paul Terry of England 'did a Marshall' – at least as far as the batting part was concerned. He had broken his arm, but came out to bat at number eleven, with his arm in a sling, so that Allan Lamb could get to his century. But who now remembers Paul Terry, gallant though he was?

The great West Indian fast bowler received the laurels for physical courage in that series and will be remembered for that reason. When Marshall was later diagnosed with colon cancer, he displayed the same pluck, slipping away almost before people realised he was ill. The hero of Headingley weighed just twenty-five kilos when he died.

Without that fortitude, if he had sought help for the stomach pains he was feeling, his condition might have been diagnosed earlier, maybe treated. But Malcolm Marshall was not the complaining type.

He may have left a few batsmen nursing bruises. But he was not found wanting when his own physical courage was put to the test. He just carried on, magnificently, without histrionics.

Denis Compton: The Brylcreemed Warrior

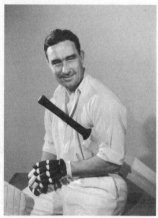

Malcolm Marshall in his pomp was such a ferocious bowler that, even now he is dead, there are probably ex-Test cricketers who wake up in the night in a cold sweat, petrified of being on the receiving end of a Marshall special.

Part of the fascination of cricket is that, unlike boxing, say, it is a form of asymmetrical warfare. If the batsman and bowler were fighting each other at close quarters, the batsman would have an inbuilt advantage: he could inflict far more damage with his bat than the bowler could inflict with the ball. But separate the two men by twenty-two yards of grass, allow the bowler a long run-up, and the equation changes.

There is a marvellous tongue-in-cheek description of cricket in *The Adventures of Brigadier Gerard* by Sir Arthur

Conan Doyle, himself a keen amateur cricketer. His French soldier-hero is captivated by the game, but for all the wrong reasons: 'There is a game called cricket, which they play in summer . . . It is a brave pastime, a game for soldiers, for each tries to hit the other with the ball, and it is but a small stick with which you may ward it off. Three sticks behind you show the spot beyond which you may not retreat . . .'

Many of the most rousing stories in cricket history date from the days before players wore protective helmets, and feature batsmen exhibiting the soldierly courage under attack that Brigadier Gerard so admired.

Whisper the words 'Compton, Old Trafford, 1948' in the ear of a septuagenarian English cricket fan and they will have the same galvanic effect as the words 'Cowdrey, Lord's, 1963' on the ear of someone of my generation. A wounded warrior battling to save his country and, in Compton's case, the Ashes at stake . . . These are mythic events, etched in the collective memory as indelibly as Agincourt or Dunkirk.

Denis Compton, the Brylcreem boy, the darling of post-war England, was an even more charismatic figure than Cowdrey. The sheer volume of runs he scored in his heyday was so extraordinary that, even in the cold print of *Wisden*, the statistics induce the same drop-jawed disbelief as the batting average of Don Bradman. 'What, you mean he scored three hundred in three *hours*?' But Compton, in his way, was an even more substantial figure than Bradman. Take away the statistics and you take away Bradman: it was as an unrivalled run-machine that the Australian left his mark on sporting history. But nobody who saw Compton in his prime dwells on his statistics. They remember the man: a professional sportsman with the heart and soul of an amateur.

And what an amateur. His amateurishness exhibited itself in a myriad of delicious ways, each more endearing than the last. He was congenitally unpunctual, often missing the start of play because he had been up all night. A ladies' man, he mislaid wives and girlfriends the way other men mislay car keys. He was a brilliant footballer as well as cricketer. At the crease, he played shots of which nobody else was capable, but when it came to running between the wickets, he was like a schoolboy playing the game for the first time. He ran out partner after partner, but they never seemed to resent it. His approach had something so haphazard about it – he would call his partner for a run and shout 'Good luck!' at the same time – that the only grown-up response was to smile. To rage at his lack of professionalism, for not getting the basics of the game right, would have been to miss the point of Denis Compton.

His demeanour on the field was so unrepentantly languid, such a glorious advertisement for cricket as a game played for fun, that it comes as a surprise to find him, at Old Trafford in 1948, playing a role more suited to a Trevor Bailey or a Steve Waugh, one of the unsmiling Roundheads of cricket.

As a batsman, Compton was at the peak of his powers. It was only a year after the 1947 season, when the Middlesex man racked up run-scoring records that will never be beaten. And in Don Bradman's Australians – the Invincibles – he had foemen worthy of his steel. In terms of raw pace, the fast-bowling trio of Ray Lindwall, Keith Miller and Bill Johnston were probably a shade slower than the West Indies pace attack of the 1980s. But with a new ball available to them after fifty-five overs, rather than the eighty of today, they were unrelenting in their ferocity. They also had a captain determined to use pace to batter and demoralise the opposition. For the Don, still scarred by memories of Bodyline, this was payback time.

By the time of the Old Trafford match, England were trailing 2-0 in the series. The gulf in class between the sides was there for all to see. At Trent Bridge, in the first Test, a tremendous innings of 184 by Compton had only delayed the inevitable. Now England, batting first, were in trouble again: 28 for two, on a lively wicket. George Emmett had been hit on the body. So had Bill Edrich. Now Compton had to face the chin music.

He had barely got off the mark when a rising delivery from Lindwall hit him on the arm. A few balls later, trying to hook a bouncer from the same bowler, he top-edged the ball on to his forehead. There was a sickening crack and, for a few seconds, the batsman staggered about the field with blood spurting from a wound above his eyebrow. He was escorted from the field, still groggy, his shirt sticky with blood. 'D. C. S. Compton, retired hurt, 4.' The scorecard in the evening papers made grim reading for English supporters.

Even after the wound had been stitched, the batsman was still feeling nauseous, and had to watch miserably as the team lost further wickets. But at 119 for five, after a quick try-out in the nets, Compton brought the Old Trafford crowd to their feet, sauntering out to bat with his head swathed in bandages. Cricket seems to provide these impossibly romantic situations more frequently than any other sport. The darling of a nation, bloodied but unbowed, putting his body fearlessly on the line.

By the close of play, after a sparkling partnership with Godfrey Evans, Compton was 64 not out, but running out of partners. His technical mastery against the fast bowling drew roars of admiration from the crowd. The Australians tried to bounce him out, but Compton played them circumspectly, defending the deliveries aimed at his ribs, ducking anything higher. Anything loose he punished, with strokes all around the wicket.

The next morning, in front of another full house, he resumed his innings in the company of Alec Bedser, reached his hundred with a sweetly timed on-drive, then, typical Compton, called Bedser for a grotesquely mistimed run. 'Sorry, partner!' By the time he ran out of partners, he had scored 145 in just over five hours at the crease.

It was not enough to win the match for his side. The Manchester weather saw to that. Yet it enabled England to have the better of a draw and, against Australia in 1948, that was as good as a win in another summer. More importantly, the innings had burnished a reputation that already shone like a beacon of hope in the drabness of postwar England.

If batsmen are the daring heroes of cricket, and bowlers the honest journeymen, it is not because batting calls for higher technical skill than bowling, but because the batsman must face such a huge range of challenges, chief among them having to fend off brutally fast bowling on unpredictable pitches. Without that element of physical danger – if the cricket ball were as soft as a tennis ball, or if only spin bowling were permitted – the game would be a dull affair. The danger gives heroism its context.

Denis Compton in his prime exuded such effortless mastery that it was easy to forget that some of the deliveries he dispatched so disdainfully to the boundary could have done him serious damage if he had missed them. After Old Trafford, vivid memories of his physical courage became an integral part of a sporting legend. The golden boy had become a golden man, with a core of steel.

Technically, there may have been better innings. Compton was dropped twice (which always means points deducted when the merits of great Ashes innings are debated). But there can have been few innings in which the fun and the fury of cricket combined to such effect.

When Compton reached his century, a Manchester dog was so excited that it ran from the cheering crowd on to the field, causing play to be held up. With a more earnest kind of hero, the comic interlude might have spoiled the story. But even a stray dog seemed appropriate in a script featuring the chaotic genius that was Denis Compton.

Rick McCosker: 'Just One of Those Things'

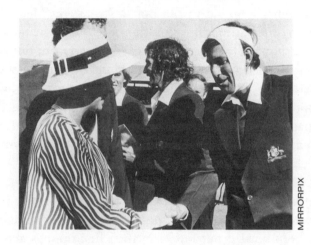

Anything an English batsman can do . . .

To bracket Rick McCosker with Denis Compton would be absurd. One was a journeyman, the other a genius. But as an emblem of courage, the batsman as patched-up warrior returning to the fray, the Australian went one better than the Englishman. McCosker's heroics in the 1977 Centenary Test in Melbourne – when he came out to bat with his head swathed in bandages, like a mummified corpse staggering from a tomb – are part of national folklore. When some wags in the crowd started singing 'Waltzing McCosker', a positively Wildean flight of wit compared with the majority of cricket chants, it put the finishing touches to one of the most lustrous legends in cricket.

The injury that the Australian batsman sustained on the first morning of the match was 'just one of those things', in McCosker's own words. It is a phrase he uses a lot in interviews and gives a clue to his laconic, matter-of-fact personality. England had put Australia in to bat, on a lively pitch, when a bouncer from Bob Willis caught McCosker, opening the batting, flush on the jaw. At first, he thought he was just badly bruised, and tried to carry on; but after losing his wicket, then being X-rayed in hospital, McCosker realised that his jaw was broken. Surgeons wired it up, then wrapped his entire head in bandages, to avoid further damage to the affected area. If common sense had prevailed, he would have been a spectator for the rest of the match.

Luckily, this being an England–Australia Test match, common sense played no part in proceedings. The stage seemed to be set for a crushing Australian victory. England had been bowled out for 95 in their first innings and, by the end of the third day, with their bowlers being flayed to all parts of the ground, were trailing by nearly 400 runs. It was not, in other words, one of those crisis situations where an injured batsman, having announced that he will bat if 'absolutely necessary', needs to gird up his loins and go out to the crease. There was no crisis, and it was not absolutely necessary that McCosker should bat. The loin-girding was unadulterated Aussie mulishness, the type that reduces English bowlers to despair. McCosker wanted to bat because, in his gritty catchphrase, 'it was just one of those things that needed to be done'.

With his baggy green cap precariously perched on top of his swaddled head, he came out to bat at the fall of the eighth wicket. Rod Marsh, closing in on a century, was at the other end. If the English fielders were surprised to see

McCosker, there was no question of them giving him an easy ride. No quarter was given, and none was expected. John Lever tested McCosker with a bouncer, which the Australian, to tumultuous applause, hooked for four. 'That's Test cricket,' McCosker said later. By the close of play, he was on 17 not out, having doggedly survived everything thrown at him.

He did not last long the next morning, falling for 25. But his partnership with Marsh had yielded 54 runs – academic, seemingly, because Australia were already so far ahead in the game, but a useful contribution all the same. McCosker returned to the pavilion to a hero's reception and prepared to put his feet up for the rest of the match.

England, set what should have been a purely notional target of 463, made an impressive fist of it, losing by 45 runs. The statisticians were in ecstasy: the winning margin exactly reproduced the winning margin in the first England–Australia Test in 1877. But that 54-run partnership between Marsh and McCosker also swelled in importance. The runs had been the difference between the two sides. No wonder the fans tumbled out into the Melbourne streets singing 'Waltzing McCosker'.

Even Her Majesty the Queen, who was introduced to the two teams in the tea interval on the final day of the match, was impressed by this soldier-like figure in bandages, looking as if he had just been patched up in a field hospital in the Crimea. In old footage of the match, you can see her give a slight double-take before enquiring after McCosker's health.

You will never get the Australian to blow his own trumpet, of course. Interviewed in 2009, McCosker was as modest as ever about what he had achieved. 'It was just one of those things you do for your team and your mates.'

That catchphrase again, like a mantra. The former Test cricketer is now an active member of his local church in New South Wales, devoting much of his time to working with young people.

His exploits at the MCG in 1977 proved historic. Twelve months later, cricket had changed for ever, not just because of Kerry Packer and World Series Cricket, but because Graham Yallop, a fellow Australian batsman, had achieved a cricketing first – he wore a full helmet in a Test match, against the West Indies in Barbados, having earlier been hit on the jaw in a tour match.

Where Yallop led, others soon followed; and A & E departments have been less busy in consequence. But the introduction of helmets also ensured that Rick McCosker, head bandaged, would be the last in a long line of ill-protected batsman heroes stretching back though Colin Cowdrey and Denis Compton to the Australians who had to weather the storm of Bodyline. They were not better cricketers, or better men, than the ones who came after them; but the uncomplicated manner in which they played the game gives them a kind of glory. McCosker and his helmetless contemporaries connect us to a world that is becoming harder and harder to imagine, but which stirs the imagination for that very reason.

Breaking a jaw was, as Rick McCosker would say, just one of those things. But playing cricket for fun, and accepting a broken jaw as an occupational hazard of that fun . . . Now that was gallantry.

Kevin Alderton: Blind Ambition

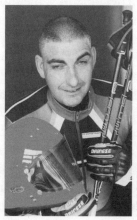

For such a universally admired quality, courage is the most personal of attributes, practically tailor-made to the individual.

Take a random list of tasks/challenges and try arranging
them in order of difficulty. For example:

(1) Eating a plateful of broccoli
(2) Flying to Venice for the weekend
(3) Delivering a speech without notes to an
     audience of two hundred people
(4) Facing a West Indian fast bowler
(5) Skiing twenty yards downhill
(6) Having a tetanus jab

Now, to most people, the majority of these so-called
challenges would not rank as challenges at all: they would

not require an ounce of courage, indeed they would be positively pleasurable to contemplate. But this is where the
idiosyncrasy of courage comes into play.

To ex-Arsenal footballer Denis Bergkamp, whose fear of
flying has been well documented, the thought of catching a
plane to Venice for the weekend, far from titillating, would
be terrifying. Likewise, there are famously fearless Test batsmen, who can take 95-mph bouncers in their stride, for
whom the prospect of having to make a two-minute speech
at their wedding is enough to bring on a cold sweat in the
middle of the night.

In my own case, challenges (2) and (3) present no terrors
at all, while even challenge (4) can be contemplated with
equanimity: after all, I would have a cricket bat in my hand
and, like all armchair cricket fans, imagine myself swatting
head-high bouncers effortlessly into the stands. But (1), (5)
and (6) are a different matter. My aversion to injections is
almost as pronounced as my aversion to broccoli and, while
I would probably plump for the injection over the broccoli,
I would have to screw my courage to the sticking point to
contemplate doing either.

But, funnily enough, it is skiing, of all the things on the
list, that most gives me the heebie-jeebies. I have seen other
people doing it and wondered where they found the nerve.
I have peered down French pistes and stayed rooted to the
spot. Even the gentlest of slopes fill me with a primal
terror . . .

. . . which probably explains my unstinting admiration
for Keith Alderton, who must be the bravest British sportsman alive.

Kent-born Alderton, 'Cannonball' to his friends, is one of
those accidental heroes who are the soul of sport. He was

born in 1971 and, at the age of eight, took his first dry ski slope lesson at Woolwich Barracks. He took to it immediately, and before he was sixteen had qualified as a dry slope instructor himself. On leaving school, he joined the Army, where he spent twelve years, serving in Northern Ireland and reaching the rank of sergeant. He also qualified as a military ski instructor and represented his unit in various Alpine skiing events.

In May 1998 his whole world was turned upside down.

Alderton and a friend had just left a pub in Islington when they saw a girl being assaulted by two men in a doorway. They rushed over to protect her, but a few minutes later, found themselves at the mercy of a drunken mob, who knocked them to the ground and started kicking them. Alderton was conscious of someone trying to gouge his eyes, but as the mob melted into the night, thought he had escaped with nothing worse than heavy bruising. Then he sneezed and suddenly the whole world went dark. He was rushed to hospital and, over the next six months, surgeons tried to restore his sight. But it was a losing battle. The soldier with a passion for skiing would have to live with just 4 per cent vision for the rest of his life. He was duly registered blind and discharged from the Army.

Alderton did not just give a philosophical shrug and get on with his life as an unsighted person on Civvy Street. Far from it. Like many of the other sportsmen featured in this book – which is what makes their stories so compelling – the skier scaled the heights of courage only after wallowing in the depths of despair. His rush to the defence of a girl being attacked was the spur-of-the-moment impulse of a decent, chivalrous man. It was quite another thing to find the reserves of patience and grit and bloody-minded determination to build a whole new life for himself.

'I had gone from being a perfectly able serving soldier,' says Alderton, 'enjoying life and doing the usual sort of lad stuff, to being without self-confidence, having no job prospects and no self-esteem. I had no motivation to carry on my life.'

For the best part of three years, he drank himself into oblivion. 'My life started to fall apart because the drink had begun to take over. Then one day I woke up and thought, I just can't do this any more . . .'

A friend of a friend suggested that he get in touch with St Dunstan's, a charitable association that helps ex-servicemen and women who have lost their sight; and the charity encouraged Alderton to go on a skiing trip to Italy in the company of Billy Baxter, the world's fastest blind motorcyclist. 'I never thought I would ski again,' admits Alderton. But coaxed on by Baxter – a fellow ex-soldier, who had also served in Northern Ireland – he slowly regained his old confidence on the slopes. Then, in a late-night visit to a bar, came the Eureka moment that changed Alderton's life.

'Billy and I were trying to think of ways in which I could get into the world record books, discussing everything from blind crocheting to blind tiddlywinks, when we suddenly just looked at each other. Speed-skiing! I was so excited that I climbed on top of the bar and announced that I was going to set the world's first-ever blind speed-skiing record at Les Arcs. People told me to get off the bar and go to bed. But I was perfectly serious. I went into training the very next day.'

With the help of Norman Clarke from the GB speed-skiing team, Alderton developed a routine that enabled him to ski downhill at speeds of which any sighted amateur would be proud. Clarke would pick out the fastest and safest line for Alderton to take, then communicate with the skier via radio speakers in his helmet, telling him to go right or left. The method was a bit hit-and-miss to begin with, but one man's unstoppable determination had made the seemingly impossible look almost commonplace.

'Courage is being scared to death, but saddling up anyway,' said that all-American icon, John Wayne. With his heroics on the ski slopes, Kevin Alderton has given new meaning to an old maxim.

'It is scary, without a doubt,' he says of blind speed-skiing, 'but I just keep practising my braking manoeuvres.' When he falls over, which he often does, it is 'as if someone has just thrown a hand grenade into a kitbag – all my stuff goes everywhere'.

In April 2006, at Les Arcs, Alderton duly realised his ambition to set a new downhill speed-skiing record for a blind person. Prefacing the attempt with a self-deprecatingly British one-liner ('You have to have a streak of lunacy in you to even attempt something like this'), he reached a speed of 100.94 mph, a figure that gets more extraordinary the more you think about it. Imagine riding a bicycle blindfold at even 10 mph. It is the stuff of nightmares.

Typically, Alderton promptly set himself new goals. 'I'd really like to reach 105 mph,' he joked. 'The current able-bodied record is 156 mph, so I'm only 55 mph behind at the moment!'

He still skis and is in demand as a motivational speaker. A life that had teetered on the verge of despair is on a steep upward slope.

'It's been a tough journey but a great one,' says Alderton. 'Hopefully, what I've done has helped change other people's lives and perceptions too.' Hurtling down ski slopes into the dark abyss is about more than conquering his own demons: it is about reaching out to others, with the same instinctive courage he showed in Islington thirteen years ago. 'If I can inspire someone to do something they would not normally do, my aims have been achieved.'

Florence Nagle: Clearing the Final Fence

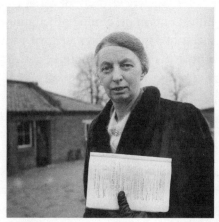

EMPICS

Timing is everything in sport. In July 1966, when race-horse trainer Florence Nagle enjoyed her fifteen minutes of sporting celebrity, the nation was so awash with World Cup fever that it must have seemed more like fifteen seconds. An epoch-making victory, one that changed the face of sport, was over in the blink of an eye.

People were too interested in the prospect of England v West Germany at Wembley to follow the case of Nagle v Feilden at the Court of Appeal. A shame. It must have been one of the most compelling sports-related cases in legal history. The cast-list alone is mouth-watering.

Of the principal men, Lord Denning, Master of the Rolls, the greatest English lawyer of the twentieth century, needs little introduction; Philip Feilden, secretary of the Jockey

Club, was an Oxford scholar and fishing enthusiast who had won a Military Cross at El Alamein; and Ambrose Appelbe, representing Nagle, was one of the great legal eccentrics, a man with a limitless appetite for lost causes. In 1935, together with G. B. Shaw and H. G. Wells, he co-founded the Smell Society, a body devoted to eliminating foul odours from London by, among other gimmicks, giving commuters sheets of paper impregnated with seaside smells.

That diminutive Florence Nagle, a retired racehorse trainer, should shine in such company says something about her feisty, never-say-die personality, brave in everything she did. At fifteen, this daughter of a wealthy English baronet had been expelled from school for driving a car without permission. At twenty-two, she had married an Irishman with a gambling problem and been threatened with disinheritance. All her life, she had been a rebel, a battler. Now in her early seventies, she had come to the Court of Appeal for justice, and she meant to get it.

Nagle v Feilden was not about an abstruse point of law or some labyrinthine dispute over stud fees. All the court had to resolve was one simple question. Could a woman train a racehorse?

There is no point in trying to turn Nagle v Feilden into a courtroom cliffhanger. The result, looking back, was a foregone conclusion. In fact, it must have been pretty much a foregone conclusion in 1966. Of course a woman could train a racehorse: it did not take the fine mind of Lord Denning to discern that. A horse could have given him the answer. The stable cat could have given him the answer. Yet it is worth recalling the uphill battle that Florence Nagle had to wage, over more than twenty years, to get the ultra-conservative Jockey Club to accept the bleeding obvious.

If one were to imagine a Sexism Steeplechase Stakes featuring those bastions of male privilege, the Jockey Club, the MCC, the Royal and Ancient, the Football Association and the All-England Lawn Tennis Club, victory for the Jockey Club would not be inevitable: one can see the R & A coming up on the rails in the final furlong. But the Jockey Club, that crustiest of patrician English institutions, founded in the mid-eighteenth century, would take some catching. By 1966, it had only got about as far as 1800 in its attitude to women. 'Get back to your knitting,' one Jockey Club member told Florence Nagle.

Far from knitting, Mrs Nagle had in reality already trained winning racehorses, and so had some of her contemporaries, including Norah Wilmot, whose owners included the Queen, and who numbered the Goodwood and Doncaster Cups among her unofficial trophies – unofficial because, in the record books, her name did not appear.

The Jockey Club preferred to maintain the fiction – one it was prepared to go to the Court of Appeal to defend – that horses trained by women had actually been trained by their stable lads. When it came to licensing women to train, the Jockey Club simply refused point-blank.

'It would not be in the best interests of racing for women to be granted trainer's licences,' the Jockey Club told Mrs Nagle, without deigning to explain or give reasons. When she pressed her case, it remained comically inflexible. 'Women are not persons within the meaning of the Rules' was another classic of Jockey Club prevarication. The heads into which Lord Denning had to knock some sense were made of solid teak.

Denning had arbitrated harder cases. 'We are not considering a social club,' he ruled. 'We are considering an association which exercises a virtual monopoly in an important field of activity.' The hypocrisy of the stable-lad fiction repelled him. 'If Mrs Nagle is to carry on her trade without stooping to subterfuge, she has to have a training licence,' he flatly told the Jockey Club.

The court found for the plaintiff and, within days, in August 1966, at a race in Brighton, Norah Wilmot became the first officially licensed woman trainer to saddle a winner in Britain. Nagle had won the argument, hands down, blazing a trail that others – Jenny Pitman and Henrietta Knight, to name but two – have happily followed.

Her victory seems so inevitable, with hindsight, that it now feels oddly undramatic, even anticlimactic, like a race won at a canter or a one-sided football match. But if you read Lord Denning's ruling in detail, you can glimpse the attitudes of the times, attitudes that needed to be challenged. 'It is not as if the training of horses could be regarded as an unsuitable job for a woman, like that of a jockey,' Denning says at one point. In 1966, post-Beatles, one of the best minds in legal history could not get his head around the idea of a woman astride a horse, competing in a race. It would be 1983 before Charlotte Brew became the first woman to ride in the Grand National.

In the ruling of Lord Justice Salmon, one of Denning's colleagues on the Court of Appeal, there is a similar note of complacency. 'No doubt there are occupations such as boxing which may be reasonably regarded as inherently unsuitable for a woman.'

In 2008 women from forty-two countries took part in the Women's World Boxing Championships in Japan. It is still a Cinderella sport, in terms of spectators, and is likely to remain so. But Cinderella, as Florence Nagle demonstrated, has her rights. You can't keep her locked up in the scullery all night. She wants to come to the ball.

Mrs Nagle died in 1988, having lived to a ripe old age. She had crammed two lifetimes into one, breeding a string of prize-winning Irish wolfhounds as well as training race-horses. It had not all been plain sailing. She had suffered divorce, bereavement, periods of penury: for a time, she had to run a teashop near Stonehenge. But her humbling of the mighty Jockey Club before the Court of Appeal out-ranks many a famous sporting victory.

Al Oerter: 'These Are the Olympics – You Die for Them'

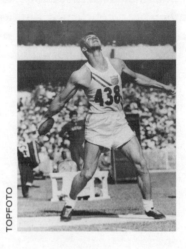

TOPFOTO

When Al Oerter was in his mid-sixties, living in retirement in Florida, the health problems that had dogged him all his life started to catch up with him. He had always struggled with high blood pressure. He nearly died in a car accident when he was twenty. Different body parts had malfunctioned at different times. To his neighbours in Fort Myers, that twenty-stone behemoth struggling along the pavement must have looked like a monument to American excess: too many hamburgers, not enough exercise.

The medical outlook was grim. Oerter, the doctors pronounced, was terminally ill with cardiovascular disease. In March 2003, he collapsed and, for a time, was clinically dead. Only a change in his blood-pressure medications stabilised his condition.

Cardiologists were now emphatic: the patient needed a heart transplant, and the sooner, the better. Al Oerter was having none of it. 'I've had an interesting life,' he told doctors, 'and I'm going out with what I have.' He did just that, dying of heart failure on 1 October 2007.

Interesting? How many of the people who saw Al Oerter in his declining years – vastly overweight, perspiring, puffing and wheezing – would have guessed that they were looking at a gold-medal-winning Olympian, by some reckonings the greatest Olympian of them all? An Olympian who had gone on to become a distinguished abstract painter?

Oerter had an interesting life all right. He was, in every sense imaginable, one of the titans of modern sport.

Alfred Oerter Jr was born in New York in September 1936. He was of German extraction and his middle name – rather inauspiciously, so soon after the Berlin Olympics – was Adolf. At high school, although he enjoyed athletics, he was far too big – six foot four and broadly built – to excel at running or jumping. Only a chance incident when he was fifteen set him on the right course.

He was practising sprinting on the running track when a stray discus landed at his feet. Without stopping to think, Oerter picked it up and threw it back. The discus went so far that it flew over the head of the boy who had originally thrown it. Oerter had found his vocation.

In 1954 he earned a scholarship to the University of Kansas, where his prowess as a discus-thrower quickly became obvious. Picked for the American team for the Melbourne Olympics in 1956, he won gold in his event. He would win gold again in Rome in 1960.

And again in Tokyo in 1964.

And again in Mexico City in 1968.

Four gold medals, in four successive Olympics, and at the same discipline. In track and field, only Carl Lewis, in the long jump, can match that record. And Oerter, in statistical terms, went one better than Lewis. Each of his medal-winning throws set a new Olympic record. He not only eclipsed his contemporaries, in other words: he redefined his discipline, continually stretching the boundaries of what was possible in his sport.

But if statistics define Al Oerter, they don't explain Al Oerter. One could put down in black and white how many metres he threw the discus each time he won Olympic gold, but, in a way, that would be a disservice to the American. His greatness as an athlete was not measurable in metres and centimetres. It lay in his never-say-die attitude: that intangible quality the record books cannot show.

Oerter was not born to courage, fearless from birth, like some athletes; in fact, he often betrayed signs of nervousness in competition, tightening up at the wrong moment. But when he had the glint of Olympic gold in his eyes, nothing could quell him. He found courage.

Perhaps the most amazing thing about Oerter, giving his unbroken run of Olympic success, was that he started every single one of those Olympics as the underdog. His rivals had thrown further than him in the build-up to the games. Or he was struggling with an injury. On each occasion he had to do something special on the day.

At the 1964 Olympics in Tokyo, where the legend of Al Oerter was cast in stone, it was very special.

The preliminaries could hardly have been less auspicious. Oerter slipped a disc in the 1963 season, condemning him to long years of back pain. In the spring of the following year, he began wearing a ski jacket to keep his body warm.

He undertook a course of ultrasonic massage and had regular injections of cortisone. He even devised a makeshift surgical collar, comprising a towel and a leather strap.

In the run-up to Tokyo, the American was not exactly fighting fit, but he was holding himself together – just. Disaster struck just six days before the discus final, when Oerter tore the cartilage in his ribcage, after slipping in wet conditions on the training ground.

For a discus-thrower, it was a hammer blow. The American team doctors were adamant that he should not try to compete in the final. They advised six weeks of complete rest. Oerter flatly overruled them. So the doctors gave him heat treatment, swathed him in surgical tape and regularly packed his right side in ice.

By the time of the final, he was in such a bad way that the simplest movement was agony. Oerter later said he felt as if someone were trying to tear out his ribs. There was no way he could win tactically, with a succession of carefully judged throws, each slightly longer than the last. He had to gamble everything on one supreme, potentially career-ending effort in the penultimate round.

He sent the discus flying, staggering out of the throwing circle doubled up in pain, in so much agony that he was not able to watch it land – an astonishing sixty-one metres away, a new Olympic record. The American had done enough. He had taken gold, condemning the world record-holder and pre-Olympics favourite Ludvik Danek of Czechoslovakia to silver.

As he choked with emotion, and grimaced in almost unbearable pain, Oerter blurted out words that have passed into sporting folklore: 'These are the Olympics – you die for them.'

Al Oerter did not, of course, die in Tokyo. He would be

back four years later, in Mexico City, taking gold, defying the odds again. But who can say what long-term damage he did to his body with his Herculean exertions in the discus ring? Unlike in many sports, which exact non-stop punishment on only some parts of the body – the knees perhaps or the ankles, or the shoulders – the discus-thrower has to contort his entire body in one spectacular, sanity-defying heave. Perhaps that is why sculptors, from ancient times, have been drawn to the subject. The throwers are putting their bodies through so much; wrenching so many muscles so far from their normal alignment. When one of them is wincing in pain before he has even picked up the discus, it is an X-rated spectacle.

Maybe that is why Oerter – in common with weightlifters and other sporting he-men – has never quite enjoyed the celebrity to which his record entitles him. Olympians with fewer medals to their name have eased him out of the limelight. People do not mind seeing runners busting a metaphorical gut as they breast the tape. With Oerter, particularly at Tokyo, the gut-busting was almost literal. It made you want to look away.

That Oerter was a man of substance, not just a magnificent physical specimen, was demonstrated after his career ended. The champion discus-thrower took up abstract painting, an interest that could be traced back to his childhood, when he was fascinated by the artwork on the walls of his grandparents' Manhattan apartment. And he proved extremely good at it. The body of a giant housed the soul of an artist.

Yet it is Tokyo, inevitably, for which he will be best remembered. In terms of raw physical courage, his defiance of the pain blazing through his entire ribcage is one of the most astonishing feats in sport.

Send in the Clowns

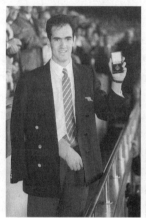

Considerate writers should respect the feelings of their readers.

The injuries suffered by Al Oerter were so gruesome that, if you are as physically squeamish as me, it can hurt just reading about them. It really can. The imagination kicks in and, as the mind ranges, you start to feel pain in the same part of your own anatomy, like the man who experiences abdominal cramps while his wife is pregnant. A feel-good sporting story suddenly becomes a feel-bad sporting story, turning the stomach more than it plucks at the heart-strings.

So perhaps, after saluting Al Oerter, it would be a kindness to take a short time out to remember some less harrowing sporting injuries.

The players involved certainly went through pain, quite

a lot of pain in some cases. They missed matches. Their careers were disrupted. They had to be rushed to hospital, X-rayed, spend hours, even days, on the treatment table. They needed to display courage, even if only the kind needed to withstand ridicule. But in the great circus that is professional sport, these are the clowns, not the lion-tamers.

Some of them made us laugh so much that we had tears streaming down our faces. Pound for pound, prat-fall for prat-fall, they provided better entertainment than many a po-faced sporting champion.

Take a very careful bow, Manchester United defender Rio Ferdinand, one of the most laid-back personalities in sport. While still at Leeds United, Ferdinand was watching television with his feet up when he strained ankle ligaments reaching for the remote control.

Goalkeeper Dave Beasant, then at Southampton, broke his foot after a jar of salad cream fell out of the kitchen cupboard. His brother, spookily, worked at the factory that had produced the guilty condiment.

Santiago Canizares, the Spanish goalkeeper, missed out on the 2002 World Cup after severing a tendon in his foot in an accident in the bathroom. Where Dave Beasant's weapon of choice was salad cream, Canizares put himself out of action with a bottle of aftershave.

Sam Torrance, the Scottish golfer, fractured his sternum after tripping over a flowerpot while sleepwalking.

Steve Morrow, the Arsenal defender, dislocated his shoulder in a freak accident after the 1993 League Cup final. His captain Tony Adams hoisted Morrow on to his back during the post-match celebrations, then dropped him like a sack of potatoes on the Wembley turf. Morrow, who had scored the winning goal, missed the rest of the season, including the FA Cup final.

Chris Lewis, the England cricketer, shaved his head before the 1994 tour of the Caribbean, then went down with severe sunstroke before the first Test in Jamaica. The *Sun* headline the next day – 'The Prat Without a Hat' – said everything that needed saying.

Alan Mullery, the former Spurs and England footballer, was forced to miss the 1964 tour of South America after injuring his back while brushing his teeth.

Lewis Moody, the beefy Leicester and England rugby player, hurt his hand one Christmas Day morning while opening presents. John Wells, his coach, called him a 'muppet'.

Alan Wright, the diminutive Aston Villa full back, strained his knee reaching for the accelerator of his new Ferrari. He later swapped the car for a Rover 416.

John Smoltz, pitcher for the Atlantic Braves, turned up at one match with an ugly red welt across his chest. He admitted that he had tried to iron his shirt while still wearing it.

Michael Stensgaard, the one-time Liverpool reserve goalkeeper, was similarly challenged in the shirt-pressing department. He dislocated his shoulder while erecting an ironing-board.

Australian cricketer Brad Hodge could iron a shirt with the best of them, but had problems lower down his wardrobe. He once missed a one-day international after injuring his back while doing up his trousers.

Step up, Alex Stepney, the Manchester United goalkeeper of the 1960s and 1970s. Stepney's team-mates included the Holy Trinity of George Best, Denis Law and Bobby Charlton. But if the goals flowed, the United defenders of that era were less dependable. Stepney had to shout at them so loudly during a match against Birmingham City that he dislocated his jaw.

Injury-prone England fast bowler Graham Dilley played a starring role in the famous 1981 Test at Headingley, but was less lucky on other occasions. He once tore a calf muscle after stopping his run-up to avoid a pigeon.

Lionel Letzi is yet another goalkeeper entitled to feel that Fate was conspiring against him. In his spell at Paris Saint-Germain, he was playing Scrabble at home, dropped a letter on the floor and strained his back stooping to pick it up. His club refused to say which letter he dropped.

Basketball legend Michael Jordan proved that even the gods of sport have failings. The great man was cutting a cigar when his knife sliced through his fingers, inflicting tendon damage.

Croatian footballer Milan Rapaic missed the start of one season at Hajduk Split after one of those little accidents to which the globe-trotting sportsman is always vulnerable. Rapaic injured his eye after inadvertently poking it with his boarding pass.

Matthew Hayden, the bull-necked Australian opening batsman, was put out of action for a time after a dog did what the England players had wanted to do to Hayden for years – bit him on the leg while he was out jogging.

Darren Barnard, the former Barnsley midfielder, was another to fall foul of man's best friend. Barnard suffered torn knee ligaments after slipping on a puddle of dog's urine.

Chris Old, the Yorkshire fast bowler, damaged his ribs after sneezing on the morning of a match.

Nery Pumpido of Argentina was the unluckiest goalkeeper of the lot, in a jinxed profession. A year after playing in the Argentina side that won the 1986 World Cup in Mexico, Pumpido was involved in a freak training-ground accident, losing his finger after his wedding ring was caught in a hook in the goal. Surgeons were later able to sew it back on.

Finally, the great, the incomparable, the rib-ticklingly funny Glenn McGrath of Australia. The man who had skittled England at Lord's at the start of the 2005 Ashes series turned his ankle after treading on a stray cricket ball in the outfield just before the second Test at Edgbaston. McGrath, who was playing touch rugby at the time, had to miss the match, which England won by just two runs in his absence, before going on to regain the Ashes. Sport has thrown up funnier injuries, but never, surely, a comedy injury with such far-reaching consequences.

It may not be quite cricket to titter at someone else when they are in pain. But where would sport be without its lighter moments, when great issues are settled by incidents of comic banality, and athletes at the peak of physical fitness succumb to accidents more appropriate to Mr Bean?

For the statistically minded, it may be worth recording that, of the most celebrated freak injuries in sporting history, more than 50 per cent have involved highly paid professional footballers.

More than 25 per cent of that 50 per cent have involved goalkeepers.

And 100 per cent of the most idiotic and embarrassing injuries have involved men.

Greg LeMond: Taking the Bullets

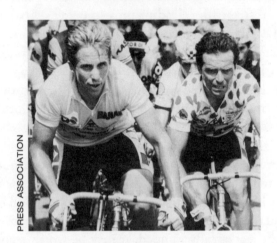

But back to the A & E department.

Shotgun wounds, thankfully, play little part in sport. As Greg LeMond not only survived his wounds, but made a full recovery, the story of how the American cycling ace was accidentally shot in the back by his brother-in-law on a turkey-shoot in California might reasonably be assigned to the previous chapter: a comedy injury, not the stuff of sporting heroism. You can bet the turkeys saw the funny side of it.

But LeMond, three times winner of the Tour de France, was a hero in more ways than one: his professional success masked underlying strains that only emerged long after his career was over.

It is not easy to imagine being Greg LeMond. Most of us

can identify with a footballer fighting cramp or a batsman getting a bouncer in the ribs: we can relate to that kind of pain. But how many of us know what it feels like to be peppered by thirty-seven shotgun pellets? Even so, it is not hard to admire the cyclist from a distance, handling himself with quiet dignity during a bucking bronco of a career.

LeMond was an oddball, a loner, more admired than loved. The comeback from cancer of his fellow American Lance Armstrong has partly eclipsed his achievements. Sport never stands still: rising stars become has-beens with terrifying rapidity. But it would be a shame if Greg LeMond were to be allowed to fade in the memory. He is a more substantial figure than that.

California-born LeMond was a pioneer in the great tradition, the first of his countrymen to win the coveted Tour de France. He won his first Tour in 1986, and could easily have won the previous year. The American was ordered to slow down by his team, La Vie Claire, so that the great Bernard Hinault, who was allegedly just behind him, could take the yellow jersey. LeMond meekly did as he was told – only to discover that, if he had not done the decent thing, he could have won the Tour himself, instead of finishing a minute and a half behind the Frenchman.

Hinault reportedly promised to reciprocate LeMond's chivalry the following year, but appeared to do little to honour his promise, according to LeMond. Relations between the two men looked strained. The American took the yellow jersey, but was fast losing his innocence. The dog-eat-dog realities of the Tour, with its labyrinthine politics and the pervasive spectre of drugs, were a depressing eye-opener for the cycling-mad kid from the States, enchanted with the romance of the yellow jersey.

But for the infamous turkey-shooting accident, which

occurred the following April, LeMond would have been
favourite to retain the jersey in 1987. Yet the cyclist was
lucky to be alive. Shot at close range by a twelve-gauge gun,
he bled profusely and survived only because a helicopter got
him to hospital in the nick of time. Even when he left hospital, his body was still riddled with pellets that it had been
too dangerous to remove. There were five in his liver, five in
his spine, and five more in the lining of his heart.

From the outside, he looked in reasonable shape, considering what he had been through. But as a professional
cyclist, he was on the critical list. He had lost 60 per cent of
his blood volume and twenty-five pounds of his muscle
mass – catastrophic in such a gruelling sport. Team cycling
can be a hard-nosed, unsentimental business. LeMond
received a get-well letter from his team, followed soon afterwards by a goodbye-and-thank-you letter. The chances of
winning further yellow jerseys were rapidly receding.

As his recuperation continued, LeMond had to be admitted to hospital for further surgery: he was suffering from an
intestinal block as a result of the gunshot wounds. At the
same time, his appendix was removed, allowing the
American to put it about that he had suffered a mild attack
of appendicitis. LeMond needed a new team to take him
on, so downplayed the seriousness of the injuries.

His return to the saddle was painful and protracted: the
weary one-step-at-a-time road trodden by injured sportsmen
the world over. He had little chance of making the 1988
Tour and, even by the time of the 1989 Tour, his ambition
was simply to finish in the top twenty. Instead, in a race that
will never be forgotten, he exceeded all expectations.

Going into the final stage, an individual time trial in
Paris, the American lay second, nearly a minute behind
Laurent Fignon of France, himself a former winner of the

Tour. It appeared an unassailable lead. But a combination of the Frenchman's overconfidence, the innovative new aerobars that LeMond was using and, last but not least, the American's bulldog spirit, secured the yellow jersey for LeMond – by eight seconds, the narrowest margin in Tour history.

He won the Tour again the next year, for good measure. And that, in terms of cementing his reputation as one of the gutsiest ever cyclists, should have been that. But there was to be a bizarre, shocking postscript. People watching the cyclist pedalling to victory up the Champs Elysees, to crown his comeback from a near-fatal injury, did not know the half of it . . .

'It appeared that everything was perfect in my life,' said LeMond, in an interview in 2007. 'It was far from perfect.'

At the height of his career, it emerged, the world-beating cyclist was carrying emotional baggage of which the world had no inkling. As a boy, growing up in Nevada, he had been the victim of persistent sexual abuse at the hands of a family friend, a malign presence in the background of his life.

'I wanted to be seen as a good person,' the cyclist says, 'and never wanted to let people down, but I found it hard to handle the fame and adulation. I didn't feel worthy of it. I was ashamed by who I thought I was, and was never able to enjoy the stuff I should have been able to enjoy.' After he had won the Tour, and become the toast of America, the spectre of the family friend returned with a vengeance. 'I thought, He's going to call. I was always waiting for that call. I lived in fear that anyone would ever find out.'

Those fears were realised in 2007 in the most dramatic of circumstances. LeMond rang his fellow American cyclist Floyd Landis, who was facing doping charges after testing positive during the Tour de France, urging him to come clean. In the course of the conversation, LeMond told the other man his own shameful secret. A few weeks later, just before he was due to testify against Landis before the US Anti-Doping Agency, LeMond received a call on his mobile phone purporting to be from 'Uncle Ron'. It was later traced to Landis's business manager, who was sacked on the spot. But, one way or another, the cat was out of the bag.

The cyclist embarked on a course of therapy and soul-searching that was infinitely more stressful than his physical recuperation from the hunting accident. 'I am now able to look myself in the mirror,' he says, with evident relief, 'and address the stuff that I was never able to address before.' He not only feels at peace with himself, but fronts a charity for the victims of child sex abuse.

Who can fail to sympathise with Greg LeMond at the moment when that Pandora's box flew open and the horrors of the past came fluttering out? And who can fail to admire the guts with which he rose to this fresh challenge?

'There are a lot of unhealthy people that are driven to sports,' he says, 'and they are driven by their own demons, their own pasts. You see it in business too. I have known some very successful, wealthy people and they are the most unhappy people you will ever meet. They can't ever get enough money. They can't ever get enough glory. They can't ever fill the hole.'

Of his own journey from the darkness into the light, he says simply: 'There was a part of me with a hole that I could never fill and it almost destroyed me. But I have been able to work through a lot of those difficulties and it feels so empowering now that nobody can hold anything over me. I don't give a **** what people say, because it really doesn't matter.'

Cliff Young: Shuffling into the History Books

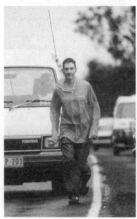

If sport has given brave men and women a stage on which to challenge racism and sexism, one should not forget the bravery of sportsmen who have challenged another of the great isms, as insidious as it is pernicious – ageism.

When golfer Tom Watson came within a whisker of winning the 2009 Open, at the quite ridiculous age of fifty-nine, it was a display of grey power to hearten anyone who had ever been written off on the grounds of age. The oldest ever winner of the Open, back in the mists of the nineteenth century, was Old Tom Morris, a venerable, white-bearded figure who looks about a hundred and twenty in the photographs, but was only forty-six, a spring chicken compared with Watson, when he won the Open for the last time.

Yet, in the ranks of the gallant elderly, even Watson must give ground to Australian potato farmer Cliff Young who, at the age of sixty-one, wrote one of the most remarkable chapters in sport. People laughed at him for taking part. He took part anyway. People said the physical strain would kill him. He refused to buckle. People said there was as much chance of him winning as of kangaroos flying to the moon. He won.

Then, just in case he was not a big enough hero already, he did something really classy . . .

Cliff Young was only a couple of years older than Tom Watson when he enjoyed his triumph, but the nature of his sport, marathon running, magnifies his achievement exponentially. Three-quarters of golf is played in the head: you need physical stamina to compete at the highest level, but it can hardly be called an endurance sport. Marathon running, by contrast, is the supreme test of heart, legs, lungs – all the body parts that start to decline once they have thirty years on the clock. As for ultra-marathons, run over hundreds of miles, they are simply not geared to old men. End of story.

Hence the mixture of scorn and bewilderment – not to mention genuine concern for his physical wellbeing – when Cliff Young pitched up at the start of the inaugural Westfield Sydney-to-Melbourne ultra-marathon in 1983. The course was one of the toughest ever to feature in competitive running, a gruelling five-day slog over 544 miles.

At first, everyone just assumed that the old man in farming overalls and gumboots was a spectator. When he joined the queue of runners getting their numbers from officials, and received the number 64, there was total confusion. Who was this guy? Was it some kind of publicity stunt?

Where was his sponsored running kit? Where were his flash trainers? More to the point, where were his teeth?

'Who are you and what are you doing?' asked a TV reporter.

'I'm Cliff Young. I'm from a large ranch where we run sheep outside of Melbourne.'

'Then you're really going to run in this race?'

'Yeah.'

'Got any backers?'

'No.'

'Then you can't run.'

'Yeah I can.'

As some of the spectators began to giggle, and the elite field, a hundred and fifty male athletes in the peak of condition, limbered up for the start, the ageing farmer with no teeth set out his race strategy to reporters.

He had been brought up on a large sheep farm in Victoria, he explained, and his family was too poor to afford horses or four-wheel drives. So, when the storms rolled in, he had to round up the sheep himself – two thousand of them, spread over two thousand acres – on foot. Sometimes he would have to run them for as much as three days at a time, going without sleep, until he caught them. And if he could go without sleep for three days . . .

Slowly the penny began to drop. This was not a stunt. It was a revolution in running. The previous consensus among competitors in ultra-marathons was that you needed to run for eighteen hours, sleep for six, run for another eighteen hours, sleep for another six, and so on. That was the most efficient way to cover the distance while conserving the necessary physical energy. At least the Cliff Young 'non-stop' strategy, albeit physically impossible and mentally deranged, had the merit of novelty.

So, inducing more giggles from spectators, did the Cliff Young shuffle. While the other runners did what runners are meant to do, and ran, Young set off from the start in Sydney at such a slow, shambling gait that it looked as though an ambulance would be needed at any minute. His arms and legs were all over the place. The man was not an athlete. He was a clown. People feared for his health. Did he realise what he was taking on? This was no fun run. It was a tough, tough ordeal.

The Young Shuffle, as it became known, has since become so popular among ultra-marathon runners that its innovative impact can be likened to the Fosbury Flop in high jumping: an apparent eccentricity that proved to be a masterstroke of aerodynamic science. Nobody was thinking about the science in 1983. They were just trying not to laugh as the old man lumbered past. Knowing Australian sports fans, they probably subjected Young to some good-humoured sledging as he shuffled through the Sydney suburbs, trailing the field, and out into open country.

Luckily, like a fair-dinkum Aussie, Young gave as good as he got.

'What's the first thing you are going to do when you get to Melbourne?' a fan shouted, when he was well into the race.

'Go to the toilet.'

The toothless old tortoise eventually beat all the sleek young hares and smashed the course record by nine hours. It still brings a smile to the face nearly thirty years after the event. His pie-eyed race strategy proved to be flawless. While the elite athletes were getting their six hours' shut-eye at the end of each day, the man used to rounding up sheep just shuffled on, and on, and on, making up the time he had lost during the day. He had no need of a trainer, or a physio, or a sports psychologist, to keep him motivated. He just imagined that he was back on the farm, trying to round up his sheep before the storm came.

As a disbelieving nation followed the race on television, the unlikeliest of sporting heroes was born: a one-off, a great original, an Australian hill-billy, the complete antithesis of the modern professional athlete. When Young crossed the finishing line in Melbourne, five thousand fans were there to welcome him. Everyone suddenly wanted to find out more about this shuffling superman who had defied time and cheated sleep. They discovered that the potato farmer was sixty-one and toothless, and a vegetarian virgin who lived with his mother and ate most of his food out of tins.

Celebrity lay in wait for Young, like a mugger in a darkened alley. The next year, like a man who has scooped the jackpot, he married a woman nearly forty years his junior. The marriage was over in five years. He still ran and, in 1997, at the age of seventy-five, tried running right around Australia, but had to give up before he had reached halfway. Nothing was ever quite the same again. After climax, anticlimax. That is always the way in sport. The magic is too good to last. As Young drifted into the sporting twilight, before dying of cancer in 2003, people preferred to remember him at the high noon of his fame, shuffling into Melbourne in 1983.

Many also remember, not only his mind-bending display of stamina and never-say-die endurance, but the little grace-note with which he crowned his day in the sun.

On being told that he had won $10,000, the exhausted farmer said he had not known there was a prize and that he not entered the race for the money. He later donated his winnings to his fellow athletes.

Who needs money? Who needs a coach? Who needs sponsors? Who needs expensive trainers? Who needs sleep?

If ever a sportsman reduced sport to its bare essentials, to reveal its nobility, it was Cliff Young.

Glenn Burke: The Man Who Gave the World High-Fives

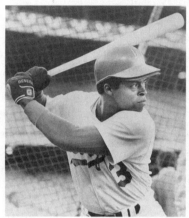

In his later years the American baseball player Glenn Burke became a tragic figure, his life blighted by drugs, homelessness and serious criminality. He died of Aids-related causes in 1995. Yet Burke is one of few sportsmen to have registered two notable firsts, quite distinct from each other and neither concerned with his sporting skills.

Burke played for the Los Angeles Dodgers and then the Oakland Athletics, and is credited with inventing the now ubiquitous high-five. In 1977, playing for the Dodgers, he ran on to the field to congratulate his team-mate Dusty Baker on hitting a home run. The two men slapped their hands together. Baker later returned the compliment when Burke hit a home run. The gesture is now seen in every team game in every country in the world.

If high-fives belong to sporting trivia, Burke's other claim to fame is more substantial. He is generally recognised as the first openly gay sportsman in a front-line team sport, a true pioneer. Homosexuality is still so taboo in sport that to have acted as Burke did in the late 1970s and early 1980s took extraordinary courage.

Born in Oakland, California, in 1952, Glenn Burke belonged to a large, poor family. His father walked out when he was one year old. At school, he proved an exceptional athlete, an outstanding basketball player and could run a hundred yards in under ten seconds. But baseball made the first call on his talents. After serving an apprenticeship in the minor leagues, Burke was signed by the Los Angeles Dodgers in 1976. By this stage, he was already openly, if not ostentatiously, gay and made no huge secret of the fact.

After his Dodgers debut, Burke was given a party at the Pendulum, a gay bar in San Francisco. Although he was well known and well liked within the gay community, admired both for his physical athleticism and for his generosity of outlook, rather than coming out fully, he maintained a discreet middle course, like millions of others, and did it with dignity.

In a perfect world, Burke would simply have told the Dodgers he was gay and everything would have been fine. The reality, according to Burke in his autobiography *Out at Home*, was very different.

Crude homophobic jokes were the accepted norm in the locker room and, although not aimed in his direction, he was painfully aware of their implications. There can sometimes be as much courage in suffering in silence as in speaking out, and Glenn Burke epitomised it.

'It was all right,' he remembered, 'but I couldn't let

anybody know who I really was. When my friends came to visit, I used to meet them in other places. I never hung out with my team-mates. In the end, I got used to the "fag" jokes. You heard them everywhere then. I knew who I was. I wasn't no sissy, I was a man. It just so happened I lived in a different world.'

'Homosexuality was taboo,' recalls Reggie Smith, who played in the same Dodgers team as Burke. 'I'm sure it would have ended his career if it had been public knowledge. Glenn would not only have been ostracised by his team-mates, but management would have looked for ways to get him off the team, and the public would not have tolerated it.'

For a time, there were two Glenn Burkes, living quite separate lives: the successful sportsman in Los Angeles and the gay man-about-town in San Francisco. 'People were just honoured to be in his presence,' remembers Tommy Lee, a restaurateur and lifelong friend of Burke. 'My God, a Major League baseball player, and he's gay! And he didn't seem to hide it. At least he didn't hide it around us. He sort of flaunted it, which was exciting.' But the strain of leading a double life was beginning to take its toll.

When the Dodgers found out about Burke's off-field activities, they took fright and offered to pay for a lavish honeymoon if the player would get married. It was not the smartest move, tactically. Burke told them to get lost. Then, more explosively, he befriended the estranged son, himself gay, of Dodgers manager Tommy Lasorda, an old-style homophobe who believed in sweeping the whole subject under the carpet. When his son later died of Aids, Lasorda told the world it was cancer.

One way or another, Burke had become too hot to handle. In 1979 the Dodgers sold the player to the Oakland

Athletics. The Oakland manager was the tough and bigoted Billy Martin, who referred to Burke as a 'faggot' and stated publicly that he did not want a gay player in the clubhouse. A year later, Burke had been driven out of the game. 'I guess the prejudice just won out,' he said, stoical in adversity.

His homosexuality only became public knowledge in 1982 through an article in *Inside Sports* magazine. Happy finally in his own skin, Burke won medals in the 100m and 200m in the first Gay Games in 1982, then competed in the 1986 Gay Games in basketball. But a year later, his career as an athlete was brought to an abrupt end when he was hit by a car. His leg and foot were crushed and he was never able to walk properly again.

By now he was also a cocaine addict, his life on a sharp downward spiral. After being jailed for theft and possession of a controlled substance, Burke was left homeless. In his final years, he became a pitiful figure, wandering Castro Street, the heart of the San Francisco gay community, asking people for money. People could barely recognise the once strong, confident athlete. He had become an aggressive, angry loser. The man who gave the world high-fives could hardly raise a smile.

Aids finally claimed the former baseball star in May 1995. Burke spent his last days nursed by his sister in Oakland, unloved, unnoticed, unmourned. Few sporting lives have ended on such a downbeat note.

'Baseball was his life,' said his mother Alice, of a life of promise cut tragically short. 'After he couldn't play any more, he felt that was the end of his life. I don't think he cared much after that.'

Glenn Burke's legacy has not been forgotten, nor has his courage.

'He was a hero to us,' said Jack McGowan, sports editor of the gay newspaper the *San Francisco Sentinel.* 'He was real. He was athletic, clean-cut, masculine. He was everything we wanted to prove to the world that we could be.'

Burke was so far ahead of his time that the changes in attitude he hoped to bring about are not even on the horizon. Not until 1999 did another Major League baseball player, Billy Bean, reveal his homosexuality, and then only four years after his retirement. Gay people may now be accepted in society at large; they are not accepted in sport, one of the last bastions of intolerance and bigotry. There is a long road for sport to travel and, the way things are going, it is going to have to be one small step at a time.

Because of his sexuality, Glenn Burke was doomed to be ostracised by his baseball peers. The most he could do was make a small statement of intent.

'My mission as a gay baseball player was to break a stereotype,' he told *People* magazine in 1994, the year before he died. 'And I think it worked. They can't ever say now that a gay man can't play in the Major Leagues, because I'm a gay man and I did it.'

Billie Jean King: Winning the Battle of the Sexes

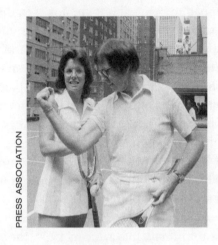

PRESS ASSOCIATION

If Glenn Burke was a tragic figure, the story of Billie Jean King, the first leading professional sportswoman to come out as gay, is altogether more uplifting.

As a standard-bearer of gay rights, King falls short of the ideal. Her admission that she was homosexual was wrung from her with obvious reluctance. It entered the public domain only when she was outed by an ex-lover in a palimony suit in 1981. There were those, including Martina Navratilova, who thought she should have been more open earlier about her sexuality.

King, born Billie Jean Moffitt in 1943, defended herself with typical robustness. 'Fifty per cent of gay people know who they are by the age of thirteen,' she once said. 'I was in the other 50 per cent.' When she married Lawrence King in

1965, she was genuinely in love with him. She became aware of her true sexual orientation only some years into the marriage, embarking on an affair with her secretary, Marilyn Barnett.

It was a furtive, covert relationship. 'I wanted to tell the truth, but my parents were homophobic, and I was in the closet,' King explained, years later. 'As well as that, I had people telling me that if I talked about what I was going through, it would be the end of the women's tour. I couldn't get a closet deep enough.'

Her account of the relationship with her strict Methodist mother rings painfully true. Every child, every parent, will be able to identify with both women. 'When I tried to raise the subject with my mother,' King recalled, 'she would say, "We're not talking about things like that", and move on.' The world-famous tennis player, who won Wimbledon six times, was stumped for a game-plan. King was over fifty before she was able to talk properly to her parents about her sexuality.

Compared with Glenn Burke, and with others in the same situation, she inched timidly out of the closet. A braver daughter might have confronted her mother earlier. But as a champion of women's rights generally, she was tireless, indomitable, someone you crossed at your peril.

For Billie Jean King, all through her professional career, winning at tennis was only part of a much broader struggle. She had a point to prove. And she proved it. Just ask Bobby Riggs.

The so-called Battle of the Sexes, contested at the Houston Astrodome on 20 September 1973, was one of those irredeemably vulgar occasions that have the real sports-lover lunging for the off-switch.

Billie Jean King entered the stadium as a parody of Cleopatra, carried aloft in a chair by four bare-chested slaves. Bobby Riggs followed in a rickshaw drawn by a bevy of scantily clad models. To the casual observer – and the event attracted a massive television audience – the message seemed clear. This was not even an exhibition match. It was a circus.

Billie Jean, we all wailed from our sofas, how could you? She had won the fifth of her Wimbledon titles two months previously. From the hallowed turf of the All-England Club to this?

Yet even in the circus, there is room for courage. King certainly needed it that day. Of all the hundreds of tennis matches she played, this was the one she could least afford to lose. To have been beaten by the obnoxious, turkey-cocking Bobby Riggs would have been a humiliation, a blow to her self-esteem from which she might not have recovered.

Riggs, fifty-five at the time of the Battle of the Sexes, was not so much an old-fashioned male chauvinist as a Neanderthal caveman. 'A woman's place is in the bedroom and the kitchen, in that order,' he once said. In his youth, he had been an outstanding tennis player. At Wimbledon in 1939, he made a clean sweep of the men's singles, men's doubles and mixed doubles titles. After the war, when he turned professional, he was ranked number one in the world. But by 1973, after the years had taken their toll, he was a pathetic has-been, making ever more desperate attempts to get publicity. His many stunts included playing tennis while holding a poodle on a leash or while tied to his doubles partner.

Riggs was sexist, vain, conceited and graceless. Taunting Billie Jean King, who was in the vanguard of women's tennis, demanding higher pay and more recognition, was grist to his mill.

'You insist that top women players provide a brand of tennis comparable to men,' Riggs told her. 'I challenge you to prove it. I contend that you not only cannot beat a top male player, but that you can't even beat me, a tired old man.'

King at first refused to take up the gauntlet, which was grasped instead by her great rival and contemporary, Margaret Court of Australia. The two women stood at the pinnacle of the sport: their 1972 Wimbledon final, won by Court, was one of the great matches of tennis. As women, they could hardly have been more different: the Australian was a committed Christian and an outspoken opponent of homosexuality. But as players, nothing separated them. So when Court took on the insufferable Riggs in an exhibition match in California in May 1973, King was a more than interested spectator.

What she saw horrified her. First, Riggs rattled Court by presenting her with a bouquet of roses before the match. As Court gave a coy curtsy, King muttered to herself: 'Margaret, you idiot, you're playing right into his hands!' Then things got really bad. Riggs, giving his opponent nearly twenty-five years, played a cunning tactical game, blunting the Australian's normally forceful attack with a series of slow spins and lobs. Court disintegrated, losing 6-2, 6-1. The arch-chauvinist had justified his boast.

It was over to Billie Jean King. Would she accept the challenge and battle to restore the honour of her sex? Or would she chicken out? The eyes of America were on her. When a $100,000 winner-takes-all match was arranged for September 1973, a whole nation rubbed its hands in anticipation.

'There is no way she can beat me,' declared Riggs, odiously self-assured. In the build-up to the match, he played every trick in the book, promising to 'psych her out of her socks'. One minute he would mock women's tennis, playing in a pro-celebrity tournament in granny rags, the next he would pay his opponent extravagant, if ironic, compliments. 'She has a better serve, more quickness, better overhead, backhand and forehand volley, more stamina,' he said mischievously. Relishing every second in the limelight, he went on a special vitamin-based diet, prescribed by an LA nutritionist, as he prepared for the match.

The lack of a reliable form-guide proved part of the fascination of the occasion. It was like a greyhound racing against a zebra: an interesting match-up, but hard to call. Yet Riggs had just trounced Margaret Court, a player of the calibre of King. One Las Vegas bookmaker made Riggs 2-5 to win. Others offered even shorter odds. As Billie Jean dismounted from her Cleopatra-style chair, and started knocking up, all the tournaments she had won around the world counted for nothing. She found herself in a dog-fight, a battle of wills, a long, long way from her comfort zone.

The result is there in the record books. King had learned from Margaret Court's mistakes and, instead of playing her usual serve-and-volley game, hugged the baseline, working her opponent around the court. She eventually won 6-4, 6-3, 6-3: not a walkover, but a comfortable, emphatic win. But it was not a victory that anyone, least of all King herself, would have predicted with confidence in advance.

She had not proved a lot in tennis terms. She could beat a man twice her age. So what? The gulf between the sexes in tennis – unbridgeable, ordained by Mother Nature – is there for all to see. In the next high-profile Battle of the

Sexes, in 1992, Jimmy Connors beat Martina Navratilova 7-5, 6-2, and that was in a handicap match – Connors got only one serve and Navratilova was allowed to hit into the doubles court.

But look at the situation counterfactually for a moment. Suppose that Billie Jean King had lost to Bobby Riggs. The damage to women's tennis would have been incalculable. The patronising jokes would have persisted, the sexist stereotypes would have been reinforced. The great goal towards which King and her fellow women players were working – equal prize money for women in the Grand Slam tournaments – would have been put back for years. Each time the insufferable Riggs opened his mouth, every woman in the country would have felt as if she had been slapped in the face.

It took a great champion taking a calculated gamble – risking public humiliation in order to make her point – to put him in his place.

Although Billie Jean may have tiptoed out of the closet, the determination with which she faced down a braggart set an example to people all over the world.

Twenty years later, there would be a touching postscript to the Battle of the Sexes, showing that, for Billie Jean King, what happened in the Houston Astrodome was not personal, but to do with deeply held principles. She had to beat Bobby Riggs. She had to rebut his patronising claims about women's tennis. She harboured no animosity towards the man himself.

The two players maintained friendly contact and, after Riggs developed prostate cancer in 1988, King telephoned him regularly. In 1995, as he lay dying, she offered to visit him, but he declined: he did not want her to see him in the condition he was. Their final phone conversation took place the day before he died, and the last words she said to him, according to King in a television interview, were 'I love you'.

Few would have seen that coming in 1973, when battle was joined on the tennis court and a feisty woman champion had to defend her sex against the forces of barbarism.

Greg Louganis: 'No Matter How I Do, My Mother Will Still Love Me'

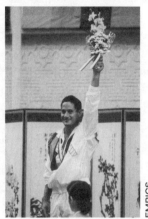

EMPICS

Greg Louganis was one of the greatest-ever Olympic divers. The American won gold in both highboard and springboard events in consecutive Olympics, 1984 and 1988. That feat alone, which has not been equalled since, would have secured his sporting immortality. But the manner of his victories at Seoul in 1988 – plus a highly dramatic sub-plot, which only emerged years later – put his courage to the severest test and made headlines around the world.

During the qualifying rounds of the springboard competition, Louganis badly mistimed one of his dives. As he went into a reverse somersault, his head caught the board, inflicting a nasty gash. The poolside crowd gasped in horror. He was bleeding profusely, and one of the Olympic doctors had to close the two-inch wound with temporary sutures: the cut would later require five stitches in hospital. Worse still, some of the blood had got into the pool.

Nobody realised – apart from Louganis himself and his coach, Ron O'Brien – that the blood-spattered diver was HIV-positive. He had been tested for the Aids virus just six months before, after discovering that a former lover was dying of the disease. To bleed so profusely, and in such a very public environment, was devastating.

'I started coming out of the dive and then I heard this big hollow thud, and then I found myself in the water,' Louganis told a TV interviewer in 1995. 'I just held my head in hope. I didn't know if I was cut or not, but I just wanted to hold the blood in, or just not have anybody touch it.'

Perhaps understandably, given the fact that it was not yet public knowledge that he was gay, Louganis had been economical with the truth before the Olympics. 'I never discussed my personal life with the media. I didn't want to make my sexuality an issue. I didn't want to be labelled The Gay Diver . . . Dealing with HIV was really difficult for me because I felt, like, God, the US Olympic Committee needs to know this. But I didn't anticipate hitting my head on the board. I didn't anticipate, you know, blood . . . That's where I became paralysed with fear.'

By his own admission, he was so stunned by the accident, and its implications, that he was too scared to say anything to the doctor treating him, even though he could see that the doctor was not wearing protective gloves. 'It would have thrown the entire competition into a state of alarm,' he explained later.

And who can blame him for his reticence? Here was a conundrum he had been grappling with for years. How, and when, to break to the world the news that he was gay? Now, suddenly, the decision was hurtling towards him, forcing him to a split-second choice when he thought he would have the luxury of finding his moment. He flunked it – as most people would probably have flunked it.

As far as the blood in the pool was concerned, Louganis could feel reasonably confident that chlorine and the pool water would dilute the virus. Medical experts later concurred: there was minimal chance of him infecting one of the other divers by bleeding into the pool. But the doctor treating him was another matter. Although the doctor would later test negative for the virus, Louganis could not know that at the time. As his wound was being stitched, the diver felt panic-stricken, guilt-ridden, paralysed with indecision.

And he still had a gold medal to win.

'Just be sure you win the damn event,' muttered his coach.

Louganis, displaying admirable coolness, took gold with something to spare in the springboard, retaining the Olympic title that he had won in Los Angeles four years before. After the accident, the eyes of the world were upon him, but he kept his composure, repeating to himself the pre-dive mantra that he always used at times of stress: 'No matter how I do, my mother will still love me.'

So far, so good. But a more daunting challenge lay ahead in the next discipline – the ten-metre highboard, the scariest, most vertiginous event in diving.

Just five years before, at a meet in Edmonton, Louganis had been a horrified spectator when a Russian diver, Sergei Chalibashvili, attempted a reverse triple somersault in the tuck position – one of the hardest manoeuvres in diving – misjudged it, struck his head on the concrete platform on the way down and plunged to his death. Ever since, the dive had been known as the 'dive of death': spectacular if executed properly; potentially lethal if not. The death of a second diver, a few years later, only added to its gruesome reputation.

In normal circumstances, Louganis would not have risked the dive of death in Olympic competition. But he was being pushed so hard by his Chinese rival Xiong Ni that, tactically, he had little option. As he prepared for the final dive, still bandaged from his earlier accident, Louganis knew that the degree of difficulty of the dive would give him a decisive advantage over Xiong – provided that he could pull it off.

In the event, he executed a near-perfect dive, left barely a ripple in the water, and beat Xiong to the gold by just 1.14 points, one of the narrowest winning margins in Olympic history. The gutsiest of gambles had paid handsome dividends.

For Greg Louganis himself, it was something of a pyrrhic victory. As he stood on the podium to receive his second medal, he was not swelling with patriotic pride, he remembers, but thinking, How soon before I get sick? What would the people cheering think if they knew that I was HIV-positive? Would they still cheer?

But from his watching coach, Ron O'Brien, who was privy to his secret, there was nothing but admiration: 'There are very few divers who could have come back from that springboard incident and won two gold medals. If that isn't courage, I don't know what is.'

Since retiring from diving, Greg Louganis has worked as an actor, written a bestselling autobiography, *Breaking the Surface*, been the subject of a TV movie, and entered his dog Nipper in agility competitions across America. The bloodied, petrified diver of Seoul is finally at peace with himself. The severely depressed teenager, who made three separate suicide attempts, is now an elder statesman of sport.

And the sport Louganis left behind has moved on, too.

At the Beijing Olympics in 2008, the gold medal in the highboard went to Matthew Mitcham of Australia, who was six months old when Louganis performed his heroics in Seoul. Mitcham was a supremely talented diver, who had come out as gay, in an interview with the *Sydney Morning Herald*, a few months before the Olympics.

Hardly anyone batted an eyelid.

The torch – of courage, conviction, nerve under pressure – had passed to a new generation.

James Braddock: The Cinderella Man

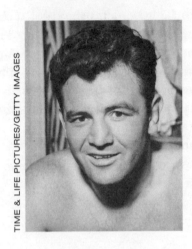

TIME & LIFE PICTURES/GETTY IMAGES

'The most courageous fighter I ever fought,' said Joe Louis. There could be no higher testimonial.

Probably the only mystery about James Braddock, most improbable of heavyweight champions, was why it took Hollywood so long to tell his story. It was 2005 before *Cinderella Man*, directed by Ron Howard and starring Russell Crowe, made it to the box office. The movie was no classic, but its story of a plucky underdog battling injury and the Depression and one of the toughest men on the planet resonated with the public. Braddock had plied his trade in a brutal, unsentimental era, but still managed to be an inspiration to millions. The 'Cinderella Man' tag was first conferred on him by Damon Runyon, that great poet of the New York underclass, who knew a working-class hero when he saw one.

Of Irish extraction, Braddock was born in the infamous Hell's Kitchen area of the city in 1905. His neighbours would have included gangsters, bootleggers, petty crooks, hard men schooled in hard times. His family later moved to the comparative serenity of New Jersey, but he never really escaped his origins. He remained, at heart, a street fighter, with the cunning of an alley cat.

Braddock was tall, just over six foot, but not as broadly built as most boxers. By his early twenties, he was a successful light heavyweight, winning forty-four of his first forty-eight bouts and earning a world title fight against Tommy Loughran in 1928. But he lost badly and, worse, fractured his right hand in several places. He soldiered on, but began to lose far more fights than he won. He had every appearance of a has-been and the Wall Street Crash of 1929 plunged him into the same penury as many of his countrymen. There was no money in boxing if you were on the losing side.

With three children to support, the boxer found irregular work as a longshoreman. At one point, Braddock had to apply for government relief money, an experience he found deeply humiliating – he later repaid the money when his fortunes improved. But temporary retirement from the ring brought unforeseen benefits. Working as a longshoreman enabled Braddock to build up his strength and physique. At one hundred and ninety pounds, compared with one hundred and seventy-five before, he was now a genuine heavyweight. His broken hand also had time to heal. He suffered from arthritis, but was a force to be reckoned with again. By 1934, he was back in the ring, written off by the boxing press, but with a burning desire to prove himself, not to mention a desperate need for cash to feed his family.

Other boxers and their promoters saw the Irishman as an easy payday. But Braddock enjoyed against-the-odds wins over John Griffin, John Henry Lewis and Art Lasky, all formidable opponents, which qualified him for a tilt at the world heavyweight title, then held by the mighty Max Baer. The fight took place in Madison Square Garden on 13 June 1935, in front of a packed, expectant crowd. As the announcer introduced Braddock, he laid it on with a trowel. 'And, making the greatest comeback in boxing *history* . . .' The stage was set.

In the movie, Baer is little more than a cartoon villain. 'You're far too pretty to be a widow,' he teases Braddock's wife, played by Renée Zellweger. But he was not just a ferocious fighter, who had killed one opponent – Hollywood, gilding the lily, stretched it to two opponents – but a complex man, capable of chivalry as well as boorishness.

By his own admission, Baer badly underestimated Braddock, and did little or no training. Braddock, for his part, was determined and focused: 'I'm training for a fight, not a boxing contest or a clowning contest or a dance. Whether it goes to round one or round three or round ten, it will be a fight all the way. When you've been through what I've had to face in the last few years, a Max Baer or a Bengal tiger would look like a house pet. He might come at me with a cannon or a blackjack and it would still be a picnic compared with what I have had to face.'

In the old newsreel footage of the fight, the difference in the two men's attitudes comes across more strongly than anything else. Baer, appreciably the bigger of the two, looks languid, even lazy. You can sense his physical power, the latent violence that made him such a feared opponent. But the body language, on this occasion, is not intimidating. He is too confident, fighting well within himself, joshing with the crowd. The Irishman, swarming around Baer like an angry insect, exudes menace and purpose. The fight went the distance, fifteen rounds, but it can have been no surprise to the spectators when Braddock won a unanimous points verdict. The world title – incredibly, after all he had been through – was his.

With the young Joe Louis, the 'Brown Bomber', waiting in the wings, he was not destined to enjoy it for very long. After Braddock had pulled out of a scheduled title defence against the German Max Schmeling – his manager was reportedly fearful that it would hand the Nazis a propaganda coup – the fight against Louis took place at Comiskey Park on 22 June 1937, in front of fifty thousand baying fans.

Braddock, thirty-two and dwarfed by the burly Louis, found himself the underdog once again. In fact, it is hard to imagine him ever being anything other than the underdog: that is the charm of his story. Unbeknown to the public, the arthritis in his hand had become so bad that he was heavily medicated, to the point that when the fight began, the drugs were acting as a muscle relaxant. He barely raised his left hand during the contest, which made him a sitting duck for the oncoming Louis. Braddock did manage to knock his opponent down early in the fight, with a fierce right hook, but was unable to capitalise and, by the eighth round, the fight was over. Some of the punches Louis threw – one of them moved a tooth right through Braddock's mouthpiece and into his lip – would have flattened a lesser man. The crown had passed to a new champion.

Braddock was magnanimous in defeat. He and Louis became firm friends and, in later life, when Louis was struggling to meet his tax bills, Braddock offered him some discreet help. But his boxing days – apart from a last hurrah in 1938, when he stopped the Welshman Tommy Farr –

were over. At the outbreak of war, he joined the Army, became a lieutenant and trained American servicemen in the Far East for hand-to-hand combat. The fighting qualities he embodied – bravery, determination, terrier-like tenacity – had never been more needed.

Hollywood, inevitably, simplified the James Braddock story. *Cinderella Man* is a sentimental, no-holds-barred homage to a decent family man battling to feed his children during the Depression. Before the Baer fight, a reporter asks the boxer what he is fighting for. Braddock has a one-word answer: 'Milk.' One misses the irony, the complexity. Do decent family men, however desperate, get into a ring and try to knock other men unconscious? The brutalities of boxing – never a comfortable sport to watch, even when it scales heroic heights – are skated over.

But to the thousands of cash-strapped New Yorkers who saved up their dimes to watch James Braddock make the comeback of all comebacks, he was not a superior mortal, a demigod. He was one of them: needy, vulnerable, dogged in adversity. Nobody better earned the tag 'the people's champion'.

Lou Gehrig: The Iron Horse

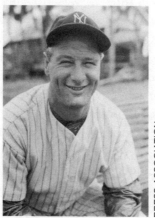

Did any sporting career come to such a poignant end as that of Lou Gehrig, the 'Iron Horse'? The legendary New York Yankees baseball star, the son of poor German immigrants, acquired his nickname because of his physical toughness. He was never injured. He never missed a match. He was not one of those sensitive flowers who are on the treatment table after the first tweak of a hamstring. He enjoyed playing baseball, so he played baseball. Between 1925 and 1939, he played an astonishing 2130 consecutive games for the Yankees. Other players picked up knocks, broken bones, little niggles. Gehrig just turned up game after game, indefatigable, his enthusiasm undimmed.

X-rays taken later in his life revealed that Gehrig had suffered minor fractures during his playing career. He simply ignored them. No other sportsman better embodied the values of the professional athlete, keeping fit, looking after himself, going about his business on and off the field with quiet competence.

As a player, even though he is often called the greatest first baseman of all time, he was probably more functional than charismatic. He was overshadowed in the Yankees team by Babe Ruth, with whom his career substantially overlapped. But, on the field, he had an aura of permanence about him: a robust, solidly built man who, for students of sporting trivia, had entered the world at a thumping fourteen pounds, the same weight as Fred Trueman, another sporting workhorse who never seemed to break down.

Then, quite suddenly, in the spring of 1939, the Iron Horse did not feel quite himself.

'I'm benching myself,' he told his manager, after a string of sub-par performances. 'It's for the good of the team.'

To baseball fans, most of them unable to remember a Yankees line-up that did not feature Gehrig, it felt like a disruption in the natural order of things. Emotional scenes greeted his omission from the starting line-up. Perhaps the great man was just feeling under the weather, jaded. He would be back for the next match, wouldn't he?

Gehrig never played for the Yankees again. Within two years, he was dead, of amyotrophic lateral sclerosis (AMS), a neuromuscular condition so rare that it is still sometimes referred to as Lou Gehrig's disease.

Had he been a fragile, injury-prone player, his sharp decline might have been explicable. In a man who was a byword for rude health, it made no sense at all. It profoundly distressed everyone who knew him. When his wife Eleanor realised the seriousness of his condition, she asked doctors not to tell her husband how bleak his long-term prospects were. 'I may need to walk with a cane in ten or fifteen years,' he wrote in the summer of 1939, oblivious to the grim medical reality.

For a time, before the disease overwhelmed him, Gehrig was well enough to work as a parole commissioner, bringing the same meticulousness to public service that he had displayed as a baseball player. But there was to be no remission from his suffering. He died at his home in the Bronx on 2 June 1941.

As flags flew at half-mast over every Major League baseball ground in America, fans were left with one last imperishable image of Lou Gehrig.

The Iron Horse was not playing baseball.

He was making a speech.

Professional sportsmen are rarely associated with oratory. They let their skills as players do the talking. But in sport it is more important than is sometimes recognised that the actors deliver their lines – congratulating their opponents, conceding defeat graciously, acknowledging the fans, all the little post-match grace-notes that send everyone home in good humour, win or lose – with skill and aplomb.

Lou Gehrig displayed that aplomb and a moral fortitude that was little short of miraculous. The setting was the Yankee Stadium, the date 4 July 1939, the occasion Gehrig's final leave-taking from the sport he had served with such distinction. Everyone knew now about his medical condition. Everyone knew that he had played his last game for the club. It was time for saying 'thank you'.

With over sixty thousand fans packed into the stadium, in an emotional ceremony held on the diamond during the Independence Day double-header against the Washington Senators, New York Mayor Fiorello LaGuardia praised

Gehrig as 'the prototype of good sportsmanship and citizenship'. His manager, Joe McCarthy, paid heartfelt tribute. Babe Ruth said a few words. The player was lavished with commemorative plaques and other gifts, which he had to put straight down on the ground – he no longer had the arm strength to hold them. Then came his turn to take the microphone.

'Fans, for the past two weeks you have been reading about the bad break I got . . .'

What power there is in simple words. Gehrig had just been diagnosed with a fatal disease so rare that there would have been more chance of him being struck by lightning while playing baseball. But he was not about to wallow in self-pity. In fact, he did the exact opposite, striking an upbeat note of such sweetness that it still sends a shiver down the spine.

'. . . yet today I consider myself the luckiest man on the face of the earth. I have been in ballparks for seventeen years and have never received anything but kindness and encouragement from you fans.'

His two-minute speech, delivered without notes, has been called the Gettysburg Address of American sport. That is hyperbole, evidently. As a phrase-maker, Gehrig was no Abraham Lincoln. But for shining courage in the face of unbearable sadness, it is a tour de force.

Humble, magnanimous, Gehrig puts self-pity to flight like a batter hitting a ball out the park. After paying tribute to his Yankees colleagues, and saying how lucky he was to have played alongside them, he publicly counts his blessings, not as a sportsman, but as a human being: 'When you have a father and a mother who work all their lives so that you can have an education and build your body – it's a blessing. When you have a wife who has been a tower of strength and shown more courage than you knew existed – that's the finest thing I know.

'So I close by saying that I might have been given a bad break but I have an awful lot to live for. Thank you.'

There was hardly a dry eye in the stadium. Small wonder that the *New York Times* the next day described his speech as 'one of the most touching scenes ever witnessed on a ball field'. And small wonder that, after his early death, Gehrig passed into baseball folklore for his human qualities as much as his playing record.

In 1942, the year after he died, he was the subject of a Hollywood movie called *The Pride of the Yankees*. Gary Cooper – who better? – played Gehrig. Babe Ruth played himself – terribly. The movie may have been on the cheesy side, but it struck such a chord with the public that it earned eleven Academy Award nominations.

In 1949, in a typically ludic poem called 'Line-up for Yesterday', Ogden Nash also celebrated the Iron Horse:

G is for Gehrig,
The pride of the stadium,
His record pure gold,
His courage, pure radium.

Like the sportsman he was, Lou Gehrig was the last man to blow his own trumpet. 'Let's face it, I'm not a headline guy,' he once said. 'I always knew that, as long as I was following Babe Ruth to the plate, I could have gone up there and stood on my head. No one would have known the difference.' But his modesty should not be allowed to disguise his greatness of spirit – or the quiet courage he showed when the eyes of the world were upon him and people looked to him to say something heart-warming, inspirational.

You have to fast-forward more than half a century to find the next time a professional sportsman spoke so eloquently in public, or found such serenity in the face of encroaching mortality.

In the pantheon of sporting orators, men who found the right words at the right moment, only Magic Johnson can be mentioned in the same breath as Lou Gehrig.

Magic Johnson: 'Life Goes On'

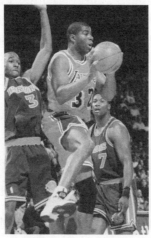

PRESS ASSOCIATION

Sharing a painful secret with one person can be harrowing. Sharing a painful secret with a roomful of journalists, in the glare of the television cameras, must be quite excruciating.

Ninety-nine per cent of the time, professional sportsmen enjoy lives the rest of us can only dream about: playing the game they love, earning silly money, basking in the adoration of fans. But when they get into trouble, when they are in the eye of the storm, when they want to hide but have nowhere to run to, the downside of celebrity becomes sickeningly clear. Is it any wonder so many crack under the pressure?

The ones who don't crack, who ride through the storm – these are the true gods of sport. And of all the sportsmen who have borne themselves with courage and dignity in the maelstrom of a media feeding frenzy, Magic Johnson surely takes the prize.

The 1991 press conference at which the great American basketball star announced that he was HIV-positive was one of those sporting occasions that transcend sport: shocking, incredibly poignant, but also, because of the impressive way the player conducted himself, oddly uplifting. It was a reminder of why sport matters – because it can change lives for the good.

Johnson only found that he was HIV-positive during a routine medical test. Jerry Buss, the owner of the Los Angeles Lakers, had wanted to give his star player a $3-million loan, but had been advised that the player would need to take out a life insurance policy as protection against the loan. Johnson, naturally, agreed.

When the Lakers' team physician, Dr Michael Mellman, saw the results, showing that the player had tested positive for the virus, he telephoned Johnson, who was in Salt Lake City for a pre-season exhibition match against the Utah Jazz, and told him he had to return immediately to Los Angeles.

The player's first reaction was of incredulity. How could he possibly have the Aids virus? He wasn't gay. His mind flew to his wife, Cookie, who was pregnant, expecting their first child. Did she have it too? As he numbly listened to Mellman telling him that he would have to retire from basketball, that he would need all his strength to fight the disease, he went into denial, refusing to accept the test results. He demanded a second test, and then a third. For more than a week, he was out of the Lakers squad, and nobody outside his family had a clue what was happening. The press were fobbed off with stories that the player had flu, or that he had a virus, and would return when he was ready. When the results of the third test confirmed the findings of the first two, there was nowhere to hide.

Early in the morning of 7 November 1991, a two o'clock press conference was called at Lakers headquarters. 'Major announcement,' the press officer told reporters. 'About Magic.'

'The announcement has to do with Magic Johnson, who has been out of the line-up since last week in Utah,' an edgy-voiced radio announcer confirmed. 'Magic could be out for a lot longer than anticipated.'

By now rumours were sweeping the city that the thirty-two-year-old star, who had helped the Lakers reach nine NBA finals and win five championships, was seriously ill. In the lead-up to the press conference, Johnson telephoned his closest friends, one after another, to deliver his bomb-shell. Then he broke the news to his Lakers team-mates, who had gathered in the dressing-room. They were devas-tated. Some were reduced to tears. Then, dressed in a suit and tie, he walked into the press room, followed by Lakers officials. There was no waffle, no beating about the bush. The gentle giant, the six-foot-nine basketball star who had charmed a nation, bent over the microphone and started talking. 'Because of the virus I have attained, I will have to retire from the Lakers . . .'

The press corps reacted with stunned incomprehension. As the news began to sink in, some journalists could be seen fighting back tears. There were no tears in Johnson's eyes: he exuded an almost Buddhist calm.

Very few sportsmen shine at press conferences, and not surprisingly. They have been taken out of their comfort zone, into the company of clever-dicks whose essential skills are verbal. Yet Johnson, though clearly nervous, was not going to fluff his lines. He was affable, even upbeat, telling reporters that he would 'beat this deadly disease'. He wanted to become a national spokesman about HIV, he said. The player, who would later admit to having had multiple sexual partners, wanted young people to understand that 'safe sex is the way to go. We sometimes think only gay people can get it, that it's not going to happen to me,' he added. 'And here I am saying that it can happen to anybody, even me, Magic Johnson.'

All kinds of questions were on the reporters' minds, some spoken, some unspoken Was Johnson really serious about retiring? Yes, he was. Were his wife and baby also HIV-positive? No, they had been tested, and were OK. How had he contracted the virus? Nobody asked. But this was not a question-and-answer session. His simple statement came straight from the heart, delivered without self-pity, with the same easy grace that Johnson displayed on the basketball court.

Through the pall of despondency that had enveloped the entire room, his sunny demeanour shone through. 'This is not like my life is over because it's not,' he told reporters. 'I'm going to live on. Everything is still the same. I can work out . . . I'll just have to take medication and go on from there.' It was almost as if Johnson were the one doing the cheering up. 'This is another challenge in my life,' he said, with a shy smile. 'It's like your back is against the wall, and you have to come out swinging.' As his confidence grew, the smile got wider and wider. 'I plan on going on, living for a long time, bugging you guys like I always have . . . You'll see me around. I plan on being with the Lakers . . . Of course, I will miss the battles and the wars, and I will miss you guys. But life goes on.'

As hard-boiled reporters wiped away tears, Johnson, dry-eyed, brought a brave speech to the bravest of conclusions: 'I'm going to go on. I'm going to beat this. And I'm going to have fun.'

The months and years that followed would introduce many more twists to the plot. Johnson came out of retirement to play in the 1992 NBA All-Star Game, and was then part of the famous American 'Dream Team' that won gold in the Barcelona Olympics. He contemplated a full return to the Lakers for the 1992–93 season, but then confirmed his intention to retire after running into opposition from fellow players, who were worried by the risk of contamination if Johnson got an open wound on court. The player briefly came out of retirement again in 1996, although he was now channelling his energies into other challenges, building up a multi-million-dollar business empire, as well as keeping his promise to promote safe sex, particularly among the young.

With the authority that came from his standing in American sport – a player who was loved and admired long before his physical condition became known – the basketball star formed the Magic Johnson Foundation to help combat HIV, published a book about safe sex, visited more than two hundred schools, made speeches at the UN, worked tirelessly to promote awareness of the disease. A sporting icon blossomed into a legend of larger significance.

President George Bush Sr spoke for millions when he said simply: 'For me, Magic is a hero, a hero to anyone who loves sports.'

The discovery that Magic Johnson had the Aids virus was a watershed in his life. Nothing could ever be the same again. But it was not, as it might well have been, a turning point of tragic moment.

At the apogee of his career, when the eyes of the world were trained on him with an intensity that few other sportsmen have ever experienced, he conducted himself impeccably and nobly. The old Hemingway line about courage being grace under pressure never felt truer.

Grant Hackett: Busting a Lung

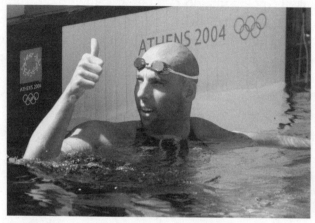

TOPFOTO

I have to admit I hesitated over the inclusion of Grant Hackett.

On the face of it, the popular Australian swimmer, revered by his countrymen, was an obvious choice for a book about sporting courage. When he won gold in the 1500m freestyle at the Athens Olympics, retaining the title he had won at Sydney four years earlier, he had to battle against a handicap that would have crippled a less single-minded competitor.

Before the final, Hackett had seemed sluggish, well below par. He was the world record-holder, but could only finish third in his heat. He was also off the pace in the 200m and 400m events. Fans started to worry.

Nobody knew it at the time – Hackett did not dare tell the team doctors – but the swimmer was suffering from a collapsed lung. He had had a bronchial infection in the build-up to the Games and, by the time of the 1500m final, one of his lungs had been become so badly blocked, with fluid in the lining, that it was partially deflated. A scan revealed that he had lost 25 per cent of his lung capacity.

Imagine going into an event as gruelling as the 1500m, one of the most challenging in swimming, with only three-quarters of your lung capacity. And imagine finding, from somewhere, the reserves of strength and stamina to win the race, against the best swimmers in the world, and set an Olympic record in the process. It must have taken a super-human effort. Yes?

Not necessarily. I don't want to rain on Hackett's parade. He is one of those effortlessly genial sportsmen it is impos-sible not to like. But buried in his story is a little subplot that gives me pause.

The lung capacity of swimmers is an arcane scientific topic, and somebody is probably writing a Ph.D. thesis about it even now. But one small statistic should illustrate its relevance. The average human being has a lung capacity of six litres, whereas the highest lung capacity ever recorded is fourteen litres, in Michael Phelps. Yes, that Michael Phelps, the American swimmer who won eight gold medals at the Beijing Olympics. Does that make Phelps a great champion or a freak of nature? You can argue it either way. But it certainly complicates his claims to heroic status.

Grant Hackett, similarly, has an estimated lung capacity of just over thirteen litres, not far short of Phelps; so even with his lung capacity reduced by 25 per cent at Athens, he would have been substantially better endowed, lung-wise, than the average person. Perhaps that superhuman feat of endurance needs to be downgraded to something a little more prosaic: a run-of-the-mill gold medal for swimming faster than the other guys.

But why spoil a good story? Sport would not be sport without myths, and if some of those myths shrink a little under forensic analysis, it would be churlish to labour the point.

One could deploy a similar argument in relation to Ian Thorpe, the 'Thorpedo', who dominated world swimming until Michael Phelps came along. Thorpe had size-seventeen feet, which gave him an inbuilt advantage. His more puny-footed rivals would have needed flippers to catch him. But how many of those rivals had to overcome the chlorine allergy – pretty lethal to a swimmer – that afflicted Thorpe when he was a boy? The lives of sporting heroes entail far more than famous wins and record-breaking times: they are made up of many chapters, every one lit by courage and determination.

Grant Hackett did not simply have to turn up at the pool, suck air into those humungous lungs, then power ahead of his rivals, as they puffed and panted in his wake. He had to train hard for more than ten years, doing far more hours of swimming, week in week out, than swimmers competing over shorter distances. He had to put his social life on hold, relocate from Queensland to Victoria, make umpteen other sacrifices, including following strict diet and hygiene regimes. The world saw a great champion. The world never saw the building blocks of his dominance in the pool.

As for bravery, physical resilience, it is easy to forget that the collapsed lung in Athens was not the first, or last, time that Hackett faced a medical setback. He suffered a bout of glandular fever in the build-up to the Sydney Olympics, when he won his first gold medal. In 2006 he had to withdraw from the Commonwealth Games in Manchester after surgery on his shoulder. Every setback challenged him in a new way.

In the twilight of his career, Hackett had to scale what some would argue is the sporting Everest – accepting a narrow, contentious defeat with grace and magnanimity. He hoped to retain his 1500m title at the Beijing Olympics, scoring an unprecedented hat-trick. He was plainly nervous beforehand, wearing a face-mask as he flew into China, for fear of inhaling something that might infect his precious lungs; but he swam a magnificent race on the day, and was beaten to the gold medal by a margin of less than two seconds. The sporting gods, for once, failed to smile on him.

'I'm not one for sour grapes,' Hackett told an interviewer after the race. The temptation was there, for all to see. Oussama Mellouli, the Tunisian swimmer who beat him to the gold medal, had just returned from an eighteen-month ban for amphetamine use. So if ever there was a time for sour grapes . . . But the Australian was too big a man to yield to temptation. He just swallowed his disappointment, and got on with his life.

In Australia, Hackett now enjoys the kind of adulation that most sportsmen, even most successful sportsmen, can only dream about. The Ferrari-owning, guitar-playing swimmer, with film-star looks and flashing smile, has endeared himself to millions. In 2007 he married pop star Candice Alley, a celebrity match worthy of Posh and Becks. In 2009 the couple announced that they were expecting a baby, then a few months later, that they were expecting twins.

And somehow even the twins seemed scripted, a variation on a theme. What would a superman like Grant Hackett be doing fathering a single baby? Shakespeare had twins. Margaret Thatcher had twins. It is only wimps who have one baby at a time. Hackett is now said to be contemplating a career in politics. They will have to build bigger ballot-boxes to hold all the votes he gets.

Vicki Moore: 'What Happened to the Bull?'

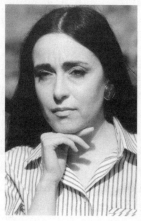

TOPFOTO

There is no point in mincing words.

If I had been brought up in Spain, brainwashed into the Spanish way of thinking, I could not have omitted bull-fighters from a book about sporting courage. The bull ring, to many Spaniards, is the ultimate in sporting machismo. It is a rarefied world, garlanded by legend, folklore, superstition. What *cojones* they have, those brave men in capes.

As I am not Spanish, and have escaped the brainwashing, I do not have to pay lip service to that vilest of sporting myths. The men in capes are not brave. They are criminals. They should be in jail. There. I have said it.

Courage in a bullfighting context is the courage to say no, to challenge age-old traditions. There are millions of Spaniards already challenging those traditions, and their views will surely prevail, perhaps sooner than we expect, as the tide of revulsion rises. But no campaigner against bull-fighting has captured the imagination quite as vividly as an Englishwoman: the late, great, Vicki Moore.

When Vicki Moore first came to attention, in 1987, the circumstances were faintly farcical. Remember Blackie the donkey? He was doomed to a squalid death, in a Spanish village where it was the custom to put the fattest man in the village on top of an ageing donkey, then drive the donkey through the streets until the poor animal expired. The story tickled the fancy of English tabloid editors who, alerted to the story by Moore, saw the chance to mount a nakedly jingoistic silly-season campaign. The *Sun* put up the money to save Blackie. The *Star* also put up the money to save Blackie. In a whirl of competing exclusives, not to mention photographers exchanging fisticuffs, the donkey was finally reprieved, then transported to a donkey sanctuary in Devon, to be patted by doting English children. And the circus moved on.

But Moore, a committed animal rights campaigner, could not, did not, move on.

Born Victoria Steel in 1956, and trained as an actress, she was working as a bunny girl at a club in Southport when she met her future husband, Tony Moore. The pair formed their own band, then got involved with the RSPCA, turning their home into a refuge for mistreated animals. After the publicity generated by the rescue of Blackie, they formed FAACE – the Fight Against Animal Cruelty in Europe – a body that is still active.

The main focus of their concern remained Spain, where the barbaric treatment of animals was widespread, both inside and outside the bull ring. In many rural areas, 'blood fiestas' were still an integral part of the social year, with animals of every kind conscripted into ritual killings and acts of cruelty, such as being set on fire, then taunted and humiliated.

In 1989, Moore used a hand-held video camera to expose another horror story from small-town Spain. For centuries, the villagers of Manganeses de la Polvorosa had celebrated the feast of St Anthony by dropping a live goat off the church tower. Once the ritual had been captured on video, the Spanish government acted quickly to ban the practice.

Yet Spanish cruelty towards bulls, in the formal surroundings of the bull ring and in traditional street festivals like the running of the bulls in Pamplona, most exercised Moore – and would eventually cost her her life.

In June 1995, in the village of Coria, doing her usual thing – posing as a tourist and taking video footage of a bull-running under cover, for fear of reprisals from locals – Moore was gored by a bull called Argentino as it was being driven through the streets. The animal tossed her into the air ten times and gored her in the chest, back, groin and legs. She also suffered a punctured lung, eight broken ribs and the loss of a kidney.

Few who witnessed the goring expected Moore to survive. But the little Englishwoman was a battler.

'What happened to the bull?' she asked, as she finally regained consciousness after a seven-hour operation. Even the Spanish press, sceptical of her motives, were impressed by her courage. 'The fleece of the lamb could not hide the teeth of the wolf,' wrote one paper admiringly. When Moore heard that the bull was called Argentino, and was alive and well, she laughed and started singing softly: 'Don't cry for me, Argentino . . .'

She spent the next five and a half weeks in intensive care

and, although she tended to make light of her injuries, was never out of pain for the rest of her short life. Despite a number of further operations, she died in Liverpool in February 2000, at the age of forty-three.

Moore had worked and campaigned right up to her death, taking her crusade against bullfighting as far as South East Asia, to the island of Macao, a Portuguese colony where it was about to be reintroduced. She never gave up confronting the evil of the corrida. She denounced it again and again and again, until people started to listen.

Like Emily Davison, the suffragette who threw herself under the King's horse at the 1913 Derby, Vicki Moore from Southport became, albeit unwillingly, a true martyr to her cause.

Millions of people feel as strongly about the Spanish treatment of bulls as she did. Since 2002, the annual running of the bulls in Pamplona has been preceded by the self-styled 'Running of the Nudes', with scantily clad women from across Europe running through the streets holding placards denouncing animal cruelty. Obviously a well-intentioned event, it always – surprise, surprise – gets a lot of press coverage. But it is not people larking about in their underwear – brave though they may be, at a banal level – who change minds, challenge the status quo, make others sit up and take notice. It is people willing to make the supreme sacrifice.

Death changes things, in sport as much as in other areas of human activity. Vicki Moore did not live to see the reforms she demanded. But she lit a torch that will not be extinguished until the barbarity of bullfighting has been outlawed.

Niki Lauda: The Better Part of Valour

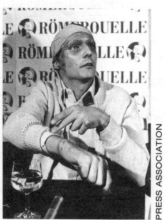

In the hierarchy of sporting courage, motor-racing drivers are at the top of the pile, higher even than boxers. Safety improvements to cars may have taken much of the danger out of Formula One, but it still has the cachet of a daredevil sport, an arena for larger-than-life heroes.

'You appreciate that it is very easy to die,' the Austrian racing driver Niki Lauda once remarked, 'and you have to arrange your life to cope with that reality.'

His own heroics in the 1976 season – combining unyielding courage with an exceptional inner calm – bore out that philosophy.

Lauda was the defending champion and not in the best physical shape. He had cracked his ribs after overturning a tractor while mowing his Salzburg property – a painful injury, but a mere flesh wound compared with what was to follow.

The Austrian surged into an early lead in the title race and, by the time of the German Grand Prix at the Nurburgring, was twenty points clear of his closest rival, the dashing English heartthrob James Hunt. Then came the accident that would define Lauda's career.

Midway through the second lap, his Ferrari swerved suddenly to the right – a rear suspension failure was later blamed – hit an embankment and bounced back on to the track, into the oncoming Surtees-Ford of Brett Lunger. Lauda's car burst into flames, but the driver was trapped in the wreckage, and other drivers, including Guy Edwards and Arturo Merzario, had to extract him from the burning vehicle. Although the Austrian was briefly able to stand up straight, it soon became clear that his injuries were serious. Hot, toxic gases had damaged the inside of his lungs; his helmet had come adrift; and he had suffered severe burns to his head. After being rushed to hospital, he lapsed into a coma and, for a time, his life was despaired of. A Catholic priest administered the last rites at his bedside.

Luckily for the Austrian, his injuries were not as bad as first feared. He suffered extensive scarring from his burns and, even today, is rarely seen in public without a red cap to cover the scars on his head. But six weeks after the crash, incredibly, he was back at the wheel, finishing fourth in the Italian GP, his head swathed in bandages from which blood was seeping. Inwardly, he later admitted, he was petrified. But the life of a racing driver had to go on.

Or did it? The sporting gods, having rewarded Lauda for his bravery, now put that bravery to the test in a dramatic way.

Although the Austrian had lost ground to James Hunt in

the title race, he was still three points ahead of the Englishman by the time of the final race of the season, the Japanese Grand Prix at Fuji. In normal conditions, Lauda would probably have won, or at least done enough to pip his rival: he was third on the grid, with Hunt second. But torrential rain threw his whole strategy into disarray.

With streams of water running along the track, and fog swirling around the course, the organisers held frantic last-minute discussions as to whether the race should proceed at all. Most drivers were in favour, but Lauda was among the dissenters, vociferously so: he thought it was mad to race in such conditions.

Outvoted, the Austrian started the race with everyone else but, halfway through the second lap, after watching the Penske-Ford of John Watson slither off down an escape lane, he pulled into the pits and got out of his car. 'My life is worth more than a title,' he later explained.

A loss of nerve as a result of his earlier accident? Or a demonstration of courage of a different kind? I know what I think. 'It is curious that physical courage should be so common in the world, and moral courage so rare,' Mark Twain once wrote. He might have had Niki Lauda in mind.

There is a time for recklessness in sport, and a time for sanity, common sense. In the gung-ho world of Formula One, the element of physical danger, for many years, was all part of the fun. The English motor-racing legend, Stirling Moss, a hero from the golden age, once likened that danger to the salt without which food would be bland and tasteless. Moss lived to tell the tale. Many of his contemporaries did not. They thought the inherent risks of their sport a price worth paying for the buzz of competing in fast cars.

Lauda, on the cusp of a new era in motor racing, took a more measured, more mature view. He did not dare the rain puddles in Fuji: he dared to challenge the status quo, which, in the long run, was far more important, not only for him, but for motor racing generally.

His decision to retire from the Japanese Grand Prix cost him the title. James Hunt finished third, good enough to take the drivers' championship by a single point. It also cost Lauda the goodwill of the Ferrari team and its all-powerful boss, Enzo Ferrari, with whom he had a major falling-out after the race. He raced for Ferrari again the following season, and won the championship with them, but then left for Brabham, before quitting motor racing to set up his own airline. Challenge after challenge, and none of them shirked.

From the time he was a boy, defying his wealthy father to become a racing driver, he was his own man, a law unto himself. He was not universally popular: people found him uptight, a control freak; he was never lavished with the same affection as more charismatic drivers. There were blots on his copybook – there are with most famous sportsmen. Charging for autograph-signing sessions was hardly the behaviour of a Corinthian. But the Austrian wrote his way into the record books by winning, and by knowing, and showing the world that he knew, when to turn his back on winning.

His dramatic shift during the 1976 season – from the fearless driver returning bandaged to his car for the Italian Grand Prix to the principled refusenik of Fuji – was one of the great chapters in sport.

Never underestimate the bravery of a conscientious objector: in the right context, it can be worth a dozen VCs.

Peter Willis: 'I Had a Decision to Make'

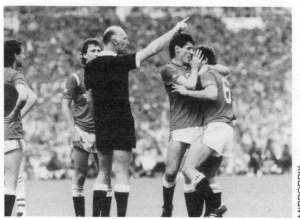

MIRRORPIX

People who enjoy football trivia rub their hands when the name of Kevin Moran comes up. First man to be shown a red card in an FA Cup final, right? Wrong! He was the first man to be sent off in an FA Cup final, playing for Manchester United against Everton in 1985. He was not shown a red card because, although a system of red and yellow cards had just been introduced, the FA in its wisdom thought that to brandish a red card would be inflammatory. I know. I was at the match.

The misconception about Moran being shown a red card has become so ubiquitous that even the footballer himself repeats the canard. 'I couldn't believe it when I got a straight red,' he told a *Guardian* interviewer in 2006. Memory can play strange tricks on a sportsman.

Even that supreme hoarder of football trivia, John Motson, believed that Moran got a red card. 'But he didn't,' I said to Motson, when I met him at a party in 2008. 'I was there.'

'So was I,' retorted Motty. 'In fact, I was commentating on the match. Moran saw red.'

'He didn't.'

'He did.'

The great man later went home, dug up his old video-tape of the match, watched it with his wife and, like a perfect gentleman, rang me to say I was right. It felt like scoring a hat-trick at Wembley.

One way or another, it was a remarkable incident, for all sorts of reasons. Irish-born Moran was a brave, uncompli-cated defender who never shirked a tackle and gave good service to club and country. But it is the bravery of the ref-eree who sent him off, Peter Willis, an ex-policeman from County Durham, that interests me.

Willis, the son of a miner, was a large, lumbering man and, as a senior referee, perhaps no better than average. One of the little oddities of the FA Cup final is that the same official never gets to referee it twice. The honour of doing it is usually accorded to a referee nearing the end of his career, as a thank-you present. It is the refereeing equiv-alent of a gold watch on retirement. Willis, officiating in his last season, was forty-seven at the time of the final. In the grand finale of his career, he was paid just £43 for his services.

But Fate was lying in wait for the Durham referee, just as it was for Kevin Moran. And what a cruel Fate, one of those acrid sporting controversies that rumble on for years. A footballer sent off in the final of the FA Cup! And for the first time! It was sporting dynamite.

From the opprobrium Willis attracted after the match,

you would think the official, not Moran, the villain of the piece. Heaven knows what would have happened to him if Manchester United had lost the final, instead of going on to win it with ten men. The club painted its player as a martyr and campaigned for him to get the winner's medal he had not been allowed to collect on the day. The FA, cravenly, capitulated. In the media, Willis got a pasting, as ex-players queued up to take a pop at him. Jimmy Greaves alleged that Willis had only sent Moran off because he was on television and wanted to make a name for himself. The referee sued and – sanity at last – was awarded damages. He gave the money to a referees' charity.

What had Willis done to become such a hate figure? How did he attract such an avalanche of criticism? It is worth trying to review the 1985 sending-off incident with the dispassion of twenty-five years' hindsight.

A disappointing game was drifting towards extra time, with the teams locked at 0-0, when a stray pass in midfield by United defender Paul McGrath was seized on by Peter Reid of Everton, who was, or would have been, straight through on goal. Kevin Moran, covering desperately, lunged in from the side, got the man and not the ball, and Reid went flying. Pandemonium broke out in the stands. The referee reached for his pocket, and everyone, including John Motson in the commentary box, thought the United player was going to be booked. Instead, after due delibera-tion, Willis sent him off. More pandemonium. Bryan Robson, the United captain, launched into a furious protest. Kevin Moran himself was so incensed that if Frank Stapleton had not restrained him, he would probably have hit the referee. It took several minutes for order to be restored.

In footballing terms, you might call it an orange-card offence, midway on the disciplinary spectrum between red and yellow. A sending-off felt harsh, given that Moran had made a genuine attempt to get the ball and had not brought down Reid deliberately. On the other hand, if he had merely been booked, the same pundits who pilloried Willis would have pronounced Moran a lucky boy. He was the last defender and, even though he was more than thirty yards from goal, his mistimed tackle had denied Reid a scoring opportunity.

'Peter Reid might have gone higher up in the air than he needed to,' Willis explained in an interview in 2002, 'but I saw what happened and I had a decision to make. I either put the whistle on the ground and walked off, or applied the laws of the game and sent Moran off . . . I've never felt guilty about it because it was the right decision to make. I just wish it hadn't happened, because I'd rather be remembered for other reasons.'

Moran disagrees. 'I didn't even think it was a foul,' he said in 2006. 'I had no intention of pulling Peter Reid down and felt I never touched him. I went into the tackle from the side and his momentum flicked him over, as if I had clattered him.'

Fans who remember the incident, or have seen replays of it, will have their own view of certainly not a clear-cut situation. You could poll fans as to whether Moran should have been sent off and the vote would probably be 55:45 or 45:55, depending on the allegiance of those voting. But one point needs underscoring. Football needs referees who have the courage of their convictions in situations that are not clear-cut.

It is easy to send a player off when he has done something that the world and his wife agree is out of order – put

an opponent in hospital with a reckless challenge or deliberately handled the ball on the goal line. It is much harder
when there is an easy get-out available, and a voice whis-
pering in your head: 'Let the boy off. Give him the benefit
of the doubt. Keep twenty-two players on the pitch.'

One of the tragedies of modern football is the extent to
which the apostles of keeping twenty-two players on the
pitch – generally ex-players themselves, with an instinctive
sympathy for players who have been harshly treated – have
been allowed to set the agenda. Such is the chorus of denun-
ciation that greets a referee like Peter Willis who errs on the
side of strictness, rather than leniency, that the arguments
for leniency – and with it, a tolerance of the professional
foul, in all its sorry manifestations – drown out other voices.
The beautiful game has become a cynical game with beautiful interludes. The lawmakers have tried to keep up with the
cheats, but been left panting in their wake.

Every defender in every league in the world repeats the
same dreary mantras to himself. *Stop your opponent by fair
means or foul. If it has to be foul means, concede a free-kick,
then defend the free-kick. If you pick up a yellow card, you pick
up a yellow card.* And for every infringement that is over-
punished, there are a hundred that go under-punished. Or
to put it another way, it pays to cheat.

Go back to that Kevin Moran lunge at Peter Reid.
Suppose he had not come flying in like that, blocking off
Reid's run. The Everton player would have been through on
the goalkeeper with, conservatively, a 30 per cent chance of
scoring. If he had scored, Everton would have been 1-0 up,
with ten minutes to play – overwhelming favourites. As it
was, even reduced to ten men, United were able to regroup,
get their whole team back to defend the free-kick, then
nick the match in extra time. The sending-off had put them

at a disadvantage, but not an overwhelming disadvantage. By that computation, it would have been a travesty of justice not to send Moran off.

So raise a glass to Peter Willis and those other men in black – occasionally pompous, inevitably fallible – who have the courage to stand up for what they believe in: a game in which attacking flair is not perpetually stifled by cynical defenders. We need them more than we realise.

After retiring from refereeing, Willis devoted his energies to the Referees' Association, of which he was president, before retiring in 2002. If you want to score a bonus point in the pub quiz, you can point out that – as authoritatively reported in the *Masonic Quarterly* – he was one of only five freemasons to have refereed the FA Cup final. The last of them was Jeff Winter, who refereed the 2004 Cup final and who once sent Alex Ferguson off during a Manchester United match against Newcastle United. And if you want to deduce from that that there is a conspiracy among the men with rolled-up trousers to do Manchester United down at every opportunity, feel free. Where would football be without its conspiracy theorists?

But it would be a shame if the qualities Peter Willis brought to football were forgotten. In the few interviews he gave, you can hear the voice of the old-fashioned copper, which is what he essentially was.

'You can't put brains there if they are not there,' he once said, 'but you can have honesty and good manners and be clean in mind and body. As a referee, I even used to say please and thank you. People might have thought I was being sarcastic, but I meant it.'

In a sport mired in cynicism, Peter Willis had the courage to stick up for the values he believed in.

Dimboola Jim: Chucking out the Chuckers

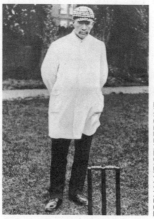

If Peter Willis risked controversy by sending off Kevin Moran, it was a storm in a teacup compared with the tempest that swirled around the head of Ross Emerson after the Australian umpire no-balled Murali Muralitharan for throwing in a one-day international in Adelaide in 1998.

'Disgraceful!' thundered Ian Botham on the commentary. The Sri Lankan team walked off the field in protest. When play resumed, and Emerson made an elementary umpiring error – in favour of Sri Lanka, ironically – his goose was cooked. The newspaper columnist Peter Roebuck branded him 'a nincompoop'. He never umpired in another international.

In a bizarre twist, it was revealed that, at the time of the

Adelaide match, Emerson was on stress-related sick leave from his day job at the Western Australia Ministry of Fair Trading. There followed snide innuendos, more mud-slinging, an acrimonious court case. And, as Muralitharan's detractors said, all because Emerson had stated the bleeding obvious. He had told it like it was. He had pointed out the elephant in the corner of the room.

Muralitharan does appear to throw. Apparently this is caused by a congenital defect in his arm. However, his critics, who are certainly not confined to Ross Emerson, believe that he throws almost every delivery he bowls. It is a nuisance. He is the leading wicket-taker in the history of the game. He is a national hero in Sri Lanka. He is a pal-pably nice man, who plays the game with a smile on his face. It is just that his bowling action is, to put it no stronger, of questionable legitimacy: unorthodox in a way that could give him an unfair advantage. What was Emerson supposed to do if he thought Muralitharan had thrown that delivery in Adelaide? Turn a blind eye? Judging the legitimacy of individual deliveries is what he is paid for.

These are very murky waters, as followers of cricket will know. At the time of the Adelaide match, the International Cricket Council, the governing body of the sport, had offi-cially cleared Muralitharan's bowling action; so Emerson, who had always thought the Sri Lankan was a chucker, and had once no-balled him seven times in a match, was acting impetuously, even recklessly, in rocking the boat. But my own hunch is that posterity, watching film footage of Muralitharan in action, is likely to see the Australian umpire as more of a hero than a villain. Like Mr Kurtz in Conrad's *Heart of Darkness*, he had something to say, and he said it.

Those steeped in the history of cricket may even find parallels between Ross Emerson and his great compatriot, the most fearless of all umpires: 'Dimboola Jim' Phillips.

In their formative years, all the major sports, and cricket was no exception, went through periods of crisis, when flawed rules had to be amended and bad practices weeded out. It took men and women of courage – many of them now lost in the mists of time – to do the weeding.

James 'Dimboola Jim' Phillips, born in Pleasant Creek, Victoria in 1860, was one of those unsung heroes. His playing career was brief and unremarkable: 1827 first-class runs; 355 wickets. He appeared just over a hundred times for Victoria and Middlesex, but never won a Test cap. He made his mark as an umpire – the first to ply his trade internationally.

Between 1894 and 1905, Phillips stood in thirteen Ashes Tests in Australia and eleven in England, earning widespread respect for his firmness and impartiality. He had the authority of someone who was familiar with cricket in both countries. In 1898, when the England captain appealed against bad light in a Test in Melbourne, after smoke from bush fires made visibility difficult, Phillips was unimpressed, joking: 'If this light is bad, then cricket had better be given up entirely at Bramall Lane and Old Trafford.'

The Australian made his most enduring contribution to cricket as an implacable opponent of 'chucking'. As the nineteenth century drew to a close, the graceful round-arm bowling that been an intrinsic part of the game had come under increasing threat from players – both fast bowlers and spinners – who had worked out that they would get better results by throwing. They had to be stopped. But how?

Sydney Pardon, the famously outspoken editor of *Wisden*, fulminated against the chuckers. Lord Harris, the *éminence grise* of English cricket, demanded that fixtures be cancelled in protest at the actions of two bowlers from Lancashire. But at the grass roots level, the cancer spread. The whole cricket world was in a dither. Defeatist voices were raised wondering whether round-arm bowling was worth defending at all. Even the great F. R. Spofforth, the 'Demon' who skittled England at the Oval in 1882, argued that the best solution might be to legalise throwing.

A large part of the trouble was that most of the umpires officiating at county matches in England were paid professionals, reluctant to bite the hand that fed them. It needed an amateur like Phillips, impartial in every sense, to stop the rot.

He first showed his mettle in Australia in 1897, no-balling the fearsome Australian fast bowler Ernest Jones, the man who once had the intrepidity to deliver a bouncer at W. G. Grace, then say 'Sorry, Doctor, she slipped', as it whistled through the great man's beard. Jones, to his great indignation, became the first bowler to be no-balled for throwing in a Test match. Twelve thousand miles away, *Wisden* thundered its approval. 'No-one who knows James Phillips can think it possible that he would have no-balled Jones without adequate cause. Nothing but good can come from what Phillips has done. If, years ago, any representative umpire had shown the same good sense, many scandals would have been avoided.'

And Dimboola Jim was not done yet.

If he thought a bowler was a chucker, he had no qualms about no-balling them repeatedly, until they mended their ways. In a match between Lancashire and Somerset at Old Trafford, he called Arthur Mold sixteen times for throwing.

Acting without fear or favour, Phillips applied his own version of zero tolerance almost a century before the phrase was coined.

Probably his most audacious decision, in a match in 1898, was to no-ball the Hon. C. B. Fry, the pre-eminent all-round sportsman of the day. Oxford-educated Fry enjoyed a standing in English cricket roughly on a par with Moses in the Old Testament, so one can imagine his reaction when he heard an Antipodean cry of 'No ball!' in his ear as he delivered the ball. His honour having been impugned, Fry offered, with glacial sarcasm, to bowl with his arm in a splint. The offer was declined.

But, if Fry was seething, the Australian umpire was winning the war. In 1900, with the tide running against the chuckers, the captains of the first-class counties held a crisis meeting at Lord's and agreed to make a concerted effort to clamp down on the worst offenders. The following year, the MCC issued a circular to the counties requesting that bowlers with doubtful deliveries should no longer be considered for selection. Some nine bowlers were duly deselected.

The nettle had been grasped – thanks largely to one man.

With his handlebar moustache, and no-nonsense manner, Phillips became a familiar figure on the county circuit in England. He was ultimately more respected than loved, probably because he did not tolerate fools gladly. After he had been criticised by a journalist for one of his decisions, the umpire confronted the man in the press box the next morning. 'And where were you sitting? Square on to the pitch? Right, I'll come and umpire the next innings from here.'

By the time of his retirement in 1906 – Phillips went on to a successful career as a mining engineer in Canada, where he died in 1930 – one hard-as-nails Australian umpire had faced down the chuckers who were destroying the English game, and emboldened others.

His mantle was taken up by Bob Crockett, a fellow Victorian, who umpired more than thirty Test matches and was nicknamed 'Chief Justice' for the meticulous way he applied the laws of the game. He no-balled one bowler nineteen times in a match, despite being jeered every time by spectators.

The spirit of Dimboola Jim lived on, fearless, unflinching.

Howard Cosell: 'I Just Tell It Like It Is'

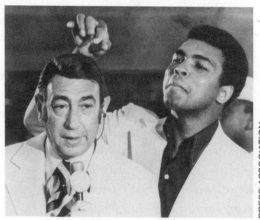

If referees and umpires have sometimes had to display exceptional courage, the same is true of that often despised species, sporting journalists. Mainly, they are just glorified cheer-leaders, occasionally booing when appropriate. But there is the odd exception.

'Let's face it,' said the legendary American broadcaster Howard Cosell, when he first got a job in sports radio. 'This is the toy department of life.' In a world inclined to take itself too seriously, his caustic good sense acted like an antidote to the hype and hysteria around him.

'The importance that our society attaches to sport is incredible,' Cosell said on another occasion. 'Is football a game or a religion? The people of this country have allowed sports to get completely out of hand.' He did not just bite the hand that fed him: he sank his teeth into it. With a tenacity that very few journalists have matched, he challenged professional sport to look at itself in the mirror. He made some tough calls in his life, but got 90 per cent of them spot-on.

Nobody would call Howard Cosell a great commentator, in the way that, say, John Arlott was a great commentator. His contributions on air were verbally skimpy to the point of self-parody. When George Foreman knocked out Joe Frazier in 1973, Cosell could manage no better than: 'Down goes Frazier! Down goes Frazier! Down goes Frazier!' His staccato delivery made him easy meat for satirists. Physically slight and unimpressive, he had a breadth and depth of intellect that was rare in his profession – dominated, as he once mordantly observed, by a 'jockocracy' of well-groomed retired sportsmen terrified of upsetting anyone.

During the 1960s, 1970s and 1980s, the one-time lawyer from Brooklyn, with his distinctive nasal twang, became one of the most familiar figures in American sport: first as the voice of TV boxing, then as a radio show host, then as an all-purpose pundit, speaking his mind without fear or favour. There has never really been his equivalent in this country. In one celebrated poll, he was simultaneously voted the most loved and most hated commentator in America. He could hardly open his mouth without upsetting someone.

A controversialist all through his life, Cosell had the arrogance and abrasiveness of the breed. But you could never accuse him of lacking the courage of his convictions. 'I just tell it like it is.' His famous catchphrase, at once cocky and self-deprecating, encapsulated the man.

Born in 1917, into a family of Polish-Jewish immigrants,

Cosell was chutzpah on stilts. He wore such an obvious toupee that it became a national joke, but was so lacking in self-consciousness that, when he was off air, he would hang the toupee on a hatrack.

His interviews with Muhammad Ali became required viewing.

'Cosell, you're a phony,' quipped the boxer, 'and that thing on your head comes from the tail of a pony.'

'You're being extremely truculent,' scolded Cosell.

'Whatever "truculent" means,' retorted a grinning Ali, 'if it's good, I'm that.'

Their relationship turned into a protracted love-in, like the similar relationship in British boxing between Harry Carpenter and Frank Bruno. But a seriousness lay behind the clowning. Ali divided the nation and Cosell, to his credit, was prepared to wade into that controversy without pulling any punches.

The world has known Muhammad Ali by that name for so long that it is easy to forget the days when he was Cassius Clay – and when his adoption of a Muslim name exposed him to ridicule and suspicion. For some years after he had taken his new name, many in boxing, including some of his opponents, still insisted on referring to him as 'Clay'. Not Howard Cosell. The broadcaster, who had been born Howard Cohen, in an age when anti-Semitism was ubiquitous, appreciated better than most that people can change their names for all sorts of reasons: what mattered was to respect them on their own terms.

His friendship with the boxer did not make him supine and uncritical – the fate of many commentators who have formed a cosy relationship with sportsmen. In 1967, when Ali infamously taunted and humiliated Ernie Terrell in a world title fight, Cosell made plain his disgust.

Whatever his personal faults – rudeness, conceit, contrariness, you name it – Cosell's moral compass was sound. 'What's right isn't always popular,' he once said. 'And what's popular isn't always right.' Later in 1967, when the New York Boxing Commission stripped Ali of his licence for refusing to fight in Vietnam, that maxim was sorely tested.

For most ordinary Americans, Ali had become a byword for a draft-dodger, reviled across the country. Cosell saw the situation differently. 'What they did to this man was inhuman,' he declared, 'and illegal under the Fifth and Fourteenth Amendments. Nobody says a bad word about the professional football players who dodge the draft. But Muhammad was different: he was black and he was boastful.'

The hate mail poured in. Cosell was damned, in his own words, as 'a nigger-loving Jew bastard'.

A year later, he was at the centre of a storm again, after the US Olympic Committee banned Tommie Smith and John Carlos for their Black Power salutes on the podium at the Mexico Olympics. Public opinion was running strongly against the athletes. 'Where will it all end?' Cosell asked sarcastically. 'Don't ask the US Olympic Committee. They're too busy preparing for a VIP cocktail party at the Camino Real.'

His decision to retire as a professional boxing commentator in 1982 was one of the bravest stances he took in his career. Cosell's disgust at the brutality of boxing welled to the surface during a protracted but one-sided bout between Larry Holmes and Randall 'Tex' Cobb, which he thought the referee should have stopped in the early rounds. Two weeks earlier, the Korean boxer Duk Koo Kim had died of his injuries after a similarly one-sided fight with Ray Mancini.

As Cobb took his punishment, and the referee, Steve Crosson, declined to intervene, Cosell posed a rhetorical question: 'I wonder if the referee is an advertisement for the abolition of the very sport he is a part of?'

Cosell got his way in the end. The boxing authorities instituted a range of reforms to the sport, reducing championship bouts from fifteen rounds to twelve and making it easier for referees to halt clearly one-sided fights. By that time, Cosell had already headed for the exit, declaring: 'I'm tired of the hypocrisy and sleaziness of the boxing scene.'

At the time, many hardcore American boxing fans saw his departure as a betrayal of the sport that had served him so well. But thirty years on, how many people would put their hand on their heart and say that the broadcaster made the wrong call? As he had done so often in his life, he told it like it was, while millions blinded themselves to the truth.

If passion is the lifeblood of sport, there also has to be room for dispassion: an awareness of the relative unimportance of winning or losing, and a sense of when, and how, to articulate that awareness.

'I don't regard myself as a rabid sports fan at all,' Howard Cosell once said. 'I couldn't care less who wins what game. To me, it's about the people, the way men react under pressure, the quality of courage.'

As to what constituted courage, the veteran commentator, who died of heart disease in 1995, was typically forthright, typically prescient. The man who had commentated on some of the most relentless fights of the twentieth century was not so profoundly in thrall to the great boxers he had known as to overestimate what they had accomplished in the ring.

'Courage takes many forms,' he reflected in old age. 'There is physical courage. There is moral courage. Then there is a still higher type of courage – the courage to brave pain, to live with it, to never let others know of it, and to still find joy in life; to wake up in the morning with an enthusiasm for the day ahead.'

His own enthusiasm for life was so astringent, wrapped up in so much Brooklyn irony, that people probably missed it. But he was one of the originals of sports broadcasting: a voice of forthrightness and sanity in a world of empty-headed cheerleaders.

Pat Tillman: When Sport Came Second

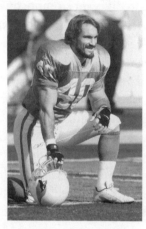

NFL

Every sports fan on the planet – not to mention millions of people with no interest in sport – knows about Muhammad Ali and his refusal to fight in Vietnam. It is probably the single best-known example of a famous sportsman doing something courageous that transcended his sport.

How many people on this side of the Atlantic have heard of Pat Tillman? At a human level, his story is even more remarkable than that of Ali and Vietnam. It combines sport, war, courage, high moral principles, an unexplained death, an establishment cover-up, and enough conspiracy theories to fill a book.

So many riddles about Tillman remain unanswered to this day that the full story of his short, tragic life will probably never be known. But we know enough about the man to accord him, without hesitation, the status of sporting hero: a man who threw down the gauntlet to his generation by raising his sights far above the banalities of winning a ball game.

Tillman was born in San Jose, California, in 1976 and, as a young man, was no different from many other young men: a mass of unassimilated testosterone looking for an outlet. 'He had this tough-guy mentality,' said his brother Kevin.

At college, he spent thirty days in a juvenile jail after a brawl outside a pizza parlour. 'I learned more from that one bad decision than from all the good decisions I have ever made,' Tillman later said.

Luckily, he excelled at sports, particularly football. Quite short, but powerfully built, with a shaggy mane of hair that gave him an intimidating air, Tillman did well at college football as a linebacker. After being signed by the Arizona Cardinals in 1998, he embarked on what promised to be a highly successful career in the NFL. In March 2002, in the middle of negotiating a three-year, $3.6-million contract with the Cardinals, having turned down a more lucrative contract with the St Louis Rams, Tillman brought the negotiations to a juddering halt.

'Hey, Frank, do me a favour,' he muttered to his agent, Frank Bauer. 'Worry about your other clients. Don't worry about me. I'm thinking of doing something else.'

The secret of the 'something else' soon emerged. Tillman, like millions of his countrymen, had been profoundly shocked by the events of 9/11, and the threat to the American way of life that the attack on the Twin Towers represented. As President Bush prepared to send troops into battle in Afghanistan, the young football player saw it as a call to arms. His grandfather had been at Pearl Harbor, but he himself, in his own words, had 'not done a damn thing as far as laying my life on the line was concerned'. Now he felt he had the chance.

In the first half of the twentieth century, such a patriotic attitude would have been unremarkable. Thousands of professional sportsmen fought with distinction in the two great wars. Hundreds – like the great Yorkshire and England spin bowler Hedley Verity – gave their lives for their countries. But by 2002 it was so long since ordinary Americans had been conscripted against their will that for a top sportsman to choose to lay his life on the line, thousands of miles from home, was a jolting corrective to the apathy and cynicism of the age.

Fame and fortune beckoned on the gridiron, but Tillman turned his back on them. In May 2002, after returning from a honeymoon in the South Pacific with his wife Marie, he told the Cardinals coach that he was enlisting as an Army Ranger, along with his brother Kevin, by now a professional baseball player with the Anaheim Angels.

It was a principled decision but, despite the high public profile the players enjoyed, an intensely private one. At the ESPN Sports Awards in 2003 – the sporting equivalent of the Oscars – Tillman and his brother were awarded the Arthur Ashe Courage Award, but did not attend the ceremony. Nor did they grant interviews. They no longer considered themselves sportsmen, but ordinary American soldiers, no different, and certainly no better, than the other soldiers in their unit.

Pat Tillman was assigned to the 75th Ranger Regiment in Fort Lewis, Washington, then took part in the invasion of Iraq in the spring of 2003, before being redeployed to Afghanistan.

He never came back.

*

The circumstances of Pat Tillman's death, on 22 April 2004, are still shrouded in the fog of war, and this is not the place to add to the mass of speculation, much of it ongoing.

The former football player died of gunshot wounds, after being shot three times in the head in an ambush near the Pakistan border. At his nationally televised memorial service a week later, he was lauded as a war hero who had died engaging the enemy. A posthumous gallantry decoration stated that he had given his life in the face of 'devastating enemy fire'. But even then the higher echelons of the military knew the truth.

The enemy had not shot Tillman: he had been the victim of friendly fire.

Disgracefully, the Pentagon came clean with his parents only some weeks after the memorial service. The Tillmans were naturally outraged. 'The fact that he was the ultimate team player and he watched his own men kill him is absolutely heartbreaking and tragic,' his mother told the *Washington Post*. 'The fact that they lied about it afterwards is disgusting.'

Tillman's father was even more outspoken: 'After it happened, all the people in positions of authority went out of their way to script this. They purposely interfered with the investigation: they covered it up. I think they thought they could control it, and they realised that their recruiting efforts were going to hell in a handcart if the truth about his death got out. They blew up their poster boy.'

A number of inquiries into the circumstances of Tillman's death were instigated. None has so far been able to reach a definitive conclusion about what happened, although the withering verdict of a Congressional inquiry published in July 2008 is worth recording: 'In the absence of specific information, it is impossible for the Committee to assign responsibility . . . It is clear, however, that the Defense Department did not meet its most basic obligations in sharing accurate information with the families and with the American public.'

By now, other uncomfortable truths about Pat Tillman had started to emerge. He may have enlisted in 2002 in a spirit of patriotic fervour, but that fervour had dimmed, to an extent, once he had seen the realities of the war on the ground in Iraq and Afghanistan.

Tillman became privately critical of the Iraq war, according to an article in the *San Francisco Chronicle* in 2005, and had urged a soldier in his platoon to vote for John Kerry in the 2004 Presidential election, when Kerry was standing against George W. Bush.

The moral complexities of the War on Terror clearly exercised the young footballer. He had thought he was fighting for a just cause, only to experience periods of doubt and disillusion. Many brave and principled Americans opposed the invasion of Iraq from the outset, the way Muhammad Ali had opposed the war in Vietnam. The courage Pat Tillman showed was of a different order. You could almost say that he was courageous twice over: in putting his life on the line for his country, when he could have stayed at home; then in looking the truth in the face, and accepting the possibility that his country might not be in the right.

He certainly gave the lie to one of the great myths of the age: that professional sportsmen are show ponies, frivolous, pampered, self-absorbed, unable to look beyond their next pay cheque.

That may be true of some sportsmen. It was emphatically not true of Pat Tillman.

Robina Muqimyar: 'Just Standing on the Track Felt Like Winning'

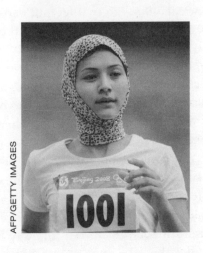

AFP/GETTY IMAGES

What was Pat Tillman fighting for in Afghanistan? There were probably times when even the footballer himself had no good answer to the question. But try phrasing it differently. Who was Pat Tillman fighting for in Afghanistan? The answer is simplicity itself: Robina Muqimyar.

In August 2004, three months after Tillman met his death, Muqimyar was part of the Afghanistan team at the Athens Olympics. There were only five in all, two of them women: Muqimyar, an eighteen-year-old sprinter, and Friba Razayee, a judoka. But their very participation was a source of joy across the sporting world. The Athens crowd cheered them to the echo as they entered the stadium.

At the Sydney Olympics four years earlier, there had

been no Afghan team, and for good reason. The Taleban had turned Afghanistan into the pariah of the sporting world by barring women from athletic competition. In fact, they barred women from just about everything. Girls like Muqimyar were kept inside the house. On the odd occasions they did venture out, they had to be covered head to toe. They received no education after the age of eight. Muqimyar wanted to run, but her ambitions were stillborn. She could only show her paces when running away from the Taleban's religious police, for fear they would catch her playing outside. Reprisals were instant and brutal, with girls and women beaten for the most trivial offences.

'There was nothing for girls to do under the Taleban,' Muqimyar remembers. 'You couldn't go to school. You couldn't play. You couldn't do anything. You were just at home all the time. As for sport, you couldn't even dream about it. You felt insecure just going outside in the street.'

After the Taleban were driven out in 2001, life took on a semblance of normality. Muqimyar attended a village school. Friba Razayee and her family, who had fled to Pakistan during the Taleban period, were able to return home. They were teenage Afghan girls who for the first time in a generation could dream of a life beyond the kitchen and the bedroom.

In 2003, when the Afghan National Olympic Committee toured the country's schools looking for volunteers, Muqimyar was the first to put up her hand. 'Other girls could run fast, too,' she recalls. 'But I had the courage.' Her 100-metres times were around fifteen seconds, nowhere near international class, and she had no trainer and no sponsor. Yet she had made a start.

The ghosts of the past were all around as she embarked on her sporting adventure. The national stadium in Kabul, where Muqimyar trained on a running track of crushed concrete, had been used for public executions and floggings. People had been hanged from the goalposts at half-time in football matches. Barefoot or in broken sandals, Muqimyar ran through this harsh space, improving her times slightly. But it was no launch pad for Olympic glory.

Before the Athens Olympics, by which time she had become the proud possessor of a pair of cheap Chinese running shoes, Muqimyar and the rest of the Afghan team trained on the Greek island of Lesbos. Given wild cards by an International Olympic Committee keen to welcome Afghanistan back into the fold, they felt the eyes of the world upon them in the build-up to the Games.

'I learned from the Taleban how to be oppressed,' Muqimyar told a reporter. 'I'm going to teach people how to be strong against them, how to learn and how to get what you want in life.'

What would she wear? That, inevitably, was one of the first questions people asked. Even in post-liberation Afghanistan, there was no question of a Muslim woman wearing the tank tops and skin-tight pants that are the norm among female athletes. Muqimyar, guided by her National Olympic Committee, sported a headscarf, a T-shirt and long green tracksuit bottoms. Aerodynamically, it was not the best choice. But who cared about the aerodynamics? History was being made.

At the opening ceremony, when Muqimyar and her fellow Afghan athletes were dressed in national costume, a telling incident occurred. As the first fireworks burst in the sky above Athens, Muqimyar gave an involuntary wince. The bangs brought back unhappy memories of the day, three years before, when she had cowered in her house while American bombs exploded in the distance.

In her first-round heat, she came seventh out of eight, just beating a competitor from Somalia. Her time, 14.14 seconds, was well short of the winning time, 11.17 seconds. But nobody was looking at the stopwatch. They were looking at this joyous young woman running her heart out, legs pumping, hair streaming behind her, raising her arm in triumph as she crossed the line.

For young women watching the Olympics on television back in Afghanistan, it must have been an extraordinary, liberating moment. But one must not exaggerate the impact of a single episode. Even after the Taleban had been expelled from Afghanistan, many of their values lingered on, particularly in rural areas.

'Some Afghan people didn't want me to take part in the Olympics at all,' recalled Friba Razayee. 'They told me I was a guy doing judo. They told me I was in big danger. They told me nobody would want to marry me.'

Political power can change hands in days. Social attitudes evolve over centuries. In the build-up to the next Olympics in Beijing, the only woman athlete chosen for the Afghan team was Mehboba Ahdyar who, according to a spokesman for the Afghan Embassy in Washington, was subjected to 'daily taunts from her more conservative neighbours, vicious rumours about her character, and even death threats from extremists'. Ahdyar went missing from a pre-Olympics training camp in Italy and was later discovered to have sought asylum in Norway.

Her absence from the team meant there was now a place for Robina Muqimyar, who had not originally been scheduled to take part in Beijing. Given the hostility that Ahdyar had encountered, she could have been forgiven for staying well away from the Games. But Muqimyar took up the place.

As a sprinter, she had regressed – her time in the first-round heat was 14.80 seconds, compared with 14.14 in Athens, and she finished eighth instead of seventh. Yet the larger statement she made was just as eloquent, just as brave, just as inspiring. Televised sport, beamed to every corner of the world, had become a stage on which the defence of freedom had found a doughty champion.

'I always wanted to run when I was a child,' Muqimyar said of the Athens Olympics. 'But I was not able to. Now the women of Afghanistan could see me and know that they could do the same. They could know they could achieve something if there was hope in their hearts. Just to go out there and stand on the track felt like winning.'

Lis Hartel: Getting Back in the Saddle

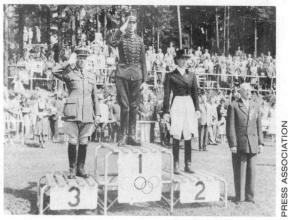

The photo of the medals ceremony after the dressage event at the 1952 Olympics in Helsinki tells its own exceptional story.

On top of the podium is the gold medallist, a middle-aged man in military uniform. The bronze medallist, to his right, is also in military uniform. Both men are giving stiff, formal salutes. There is no such formality about the silver medallist, a young woman in white jodhpurs, dark jacket and black hat. She has a handkerchief in her hand and is wiping away a tear.

Lis Hartel of Denmark, horse-mad since she was a child, had just broken into one of the most tightly closed shops in sport, finishing runner-up in the dressage on her beloved horse Jubilee. There had been equestrian events at every

Olympics since the Stockholm Games in 1912, but they were open only to cavalry officers, which eliminated Hartel at the first fence. She was as good at dressage as any man – she became Danish national champion at the age of just twenty-two – but found her path to Olympic glory blocked by the dead hand of custom and tradition. To the diehards of the equestrian world, dressage was not a sport, but an esoteric horse ballet performed by officers and gentlemen.

At the London Olympics in 1948 – in an incident that well illustrates the cultural attitudes that Hartel was challenging – the entire Swedish dressage team was disqualified and stripped of its gold medal after officials discovered that one of its team members was a non-commissioned officer. The shame of it!

Even at Helsinki, where women were grudgingly admitted into the dressage, they remained strictly excluded from the eventing and the show-jumping. Old prejudices die hard. Presumably the International Olympic Committee had seen women riding horses before: they had just not been able to make the necessary connection between women on horseback and equestrian competition.

At least now, thanks to Lis Hartel, women had got a foot in the door – and a silver medal too.

Well might such a pioneer allow herself a quiet tear on the podium.

But to get on that podium the Danish rider had to overcome a far greater handicap than being a woman.

The stiffness of her legs in the picture gives the game away. Lis Hartel had had polio – like many people in the pre-vaccination era – and her legs were paralysed below the knees. That she was riding a horse at all, never mind taking the silver medal, was a miracle.

The disease had struck in 1944, when Hartel was twenty-three and pregnant with her first child. It left her, she recalled later, 'almost entirely paralysed'. Already Danish dressage champion, she was utterly determined to resume her riding career. That meant beginning rehabilitation at once and continuing after she had delivered her child. It was a long battle, excruciatingly slow. She had to learn to lift her arms again, then to crawl, then to try and walk. Every step on the journey was agony.

Most sporting events are over in a matter of hours. We cheer on our favourites, then go home elated or disappointed, depending on whether they have won or lost. We rarely see the behind-the-scenes drudgery: the hours of practice, the gruelling training regimes, the almost superhuman sacrifices. When we glimpse that world of aching bones and gritted teeth, as we are able to do in the case of Lis Hartel, it is inspiring and humbling.

Learning to crawl proved the hardest part of her rehabilitation. It was like reverting to infancy. She would lie face down on the floor, with a towel under her body, held by her husband and her mother. As they lifted her slightly from the floor, she would try to crawl forward. After a matter of inches, she became exhausted. By the time she was put to bed, she had reached a state of near collapse. Hartel set herself the goal of crawling a yard further every day until she had regained the use of her muscles.

Learning to walk would be similarly painful. It took eight months for her to progress from walking on crutches to the point where she could hobble along with the help of two canes.

Resuming her career in the saddle presented the final challenge. At first, for Hartel and her family, it felt like a bridge too far. She toppled off her horse repeatedly, collapsed from exhaustion again and again, and came close to giving up. But, although she remained partly paralysed in her left side and had limited use of her hands, she gradually regained the use of her thigh muscles sufficiently to keep her seat at a trot. By 1947, just three years after the polio attack, she was competing in the Scandinavian championships, finishing second.

Physically, Hartel was still impaired. She had to be helped on to her horse every time she rode. When she won the silver medal at Helsinki, the gold medallist, Henri Saint Cyr, had to lift her on to the podium, providing one of the abiding images of the Games. But she was back doing what she did best and, in one of the few sports at which men and women compete on equal terms, challenging for the highest honours, continuing to win national championships throughout the 1950s.

At the Melbourne Olympics in 1956, because of quarantine laws, the equestrian events were held in Stockholm, which was a lucky break for the Danish rider. She won the silver medal again, proving that Helsinki was no sentimental flash in the pan, before retiring from Olympic competition.

But not – and this is one of the most touching features of the Lis Hartel story – retiring from sport altogether.

Right up to her death in 2009, at the age of eighty-seven, the Danish dressage champion was actively involved in helping other disabled riders benefit from her experience and know-how. As a girl, she had taken up riding for the simplest and purest of reasons: because it was fun. As a woman, schooled in the severest adversity, she had learned that it could also be therapeutic: a stepping-stone from disappointment and self-doubt to a fuller emotional life.

How often when that old cliché comes tumbling out – 'I

want to give something back' – does one glimpse a largely selfish agenda? Many a sportsman spouting the cliché is not primarily interested in giving: he wants to bolster his income post-retirement. Not Lis Hartel.

After retiring from competition, she travelled the world giving demonstrations, raising money for polio and championing the cause of therapeutic riding for the disabled. Thanks to her example, there are now Riding for the Disabled associations as far afield as Dubai and Australia, as well as the Lis Hartel Foundation in the Netherlands, a charity dedicated to offering riding opportunities to people with disabilities.

Her legacy to her sport is more intangible than medals in a trophy cabinet. It is a faith in the possibility of joy.

Wilma Rudolph: Defying the Odds

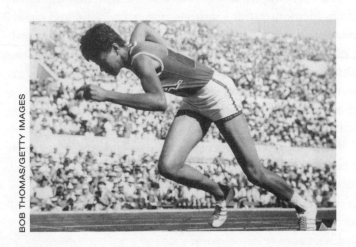

Lis Hartel's heroic battle with polio recalls the exploits of another great Olympian: the American sprinter Wilma Rudolph. At the Rome Olympics in 1960, despite a slight ankle strain, Rudolph pulled off the classic sprinter's hat-trick: gold medals in the 100m, 200m and 4 × 100m relay. The Italians were so enchanted by the twenty-year-old from Tennessee, smashing records right, left and centre, that they nicknamed her 'The Black Gazelle'. Her absolute mastery on the track made it hard to believe that as a small child, struck down with polio, Rudolph had been so sick doctors had said she would never walk unaided again.

Her own account of her childhood has a charming simplicity, an inspiring human epic told in three sentences:

'The doctors told me I would never walk again. My mother told me I would. I believed my mother.'

Battling the odds had been ingrained in Rudolph from the first day she drew breath, on 23 June 1940 in Clarksville, Tennessee, the seventeenth of nineteen children. Her father was a railroad porter and handyman. Her mother did cooking and cleaning for wealthy white families. Wilma, born two months prematurely, weighed four and a half pounds at birth. She was lucky to survive. Babies born that underweight in Tennessee in the early 1940s were given only a fifty-fifty chance. For black babies, in what was still a strictly segregated state, the odds were much longer.

For most of her early years, Rudolph was sickly, housebound, afflicted by one illness after another. She did not attend the local, segregated, school until the age of seven. Not that studies were uppermost in her mind. She had already been diagnosed with infantile paralysis, as a result of polio. Scarlet fever, whooping cough, chicken pox, measles and double pneumonia followed in debilitating succession. The nearest hospital – the nearest that would treat blacks – was a fifty-mile bus ride away.

At seven, Rudolph was still wearing a leg brace and a corrective shoe. Doctors, more in hope than expectation, recommended a routine of massage for her affected leg. They underestimated the reserves of determination in the sickly child and the human support systems at work in a large family. Rudolph got the four-times-a-day massages she needed from her mother and father, and from her elder siblings. 'No matter what accomplishments you make,' she said, years later, 'somebody helps you.'

By the time she was nine, the leg brace had been discarded. By the age of eleven, the corrective shoe had followed, and Rudolph was playing basketball in the yard with her brothers. At thirteen, she was the fastest girl in the neighbourhood, so fast that people started to see her, not simply as a former polio-sufferer who had done well for herself, but as a potential champion.

Ed Temple, the track coach at Tennessee State University, certainly recognised talent when he saw it. The young sprinter made such giant strides under his tutelage that, at the age of sixteen, she was flying to Melbourne as part of the American 4 × 100m relay team at the 1956 Olympics. The team managed to win only bronze, but a first Olympic medal for Rudolph whetted her appetite for more. Soon she began training with the famous Tigerbelles, the elite women's athletic squad at Tennessee State University.

It was not all plain sailing. Rudolph had to miss most of the 1958 season as the rigours of top-flight athletics took their toll. But the flame of ambition had been lit. Rudolph did not only want to be the fastest woman on the planet: she wanted to emulate Jesse Owens, her sporting idol, who had won triple gold at the Berlin Olympics in 1936 and been an inspiration to black athletes all over the world.

'Never underestimate the power of dreams and the influence of the human spirit,' Rudolph once said. 'The potential for greatness lies within each of us.' She was about to liberate that potential in the most spectacular fashion, turning in just four years from promising teenager to world-beater.

One of her other favourite maxims was that 'the triumph could not be had without the struggle'. All her life had been a struggle: now, on the running track, that struggle had a sharper focus. Sprinters can sometimes seem like the athletes who have to train least hard, the ones born with natural ability who simply have to unleash that ability on the track. Wilma Rudolph's account of her road to Olympic glory gives the lie to that perception.

'I ran and ran every day,' she remembered, 'and I acquired this sense of determination, this sense of spirit that I would never, never give up, no matter what happened.'

By the time she arrived in Rome for the 1960 Olympics, she was not in absolutely top condition: an ankle strain had hampered her preparations. But she still ran far too fast for the competition, winning both the 100m and 200m finals with something to spare. In the 4 × 100m relay final she needed to demonstrate her never-say-die spirit, helping the Americans come from behind to win, after a clumsy baton handover.

In a few sunlit days in the Eternal City, Wilma Rudolph's great dream of becoming the female Jesse Owens had become reality. But her work was not finished. It never is with a champion athlete. There are new targets, new challenges. And they are not necessarily confined to sport.

In 1936, when Jesse Owens returned in triumph from Berlin, America was not ready to embrace a black athlete with open arms. The habits of racial discrimination were too ingrained. There was no welcome to the White House from Franklin D. Roosevelt. Owens received a tickertape reception in New York but, disgracefully, had to take the service lift to the party held in his honour at the Waldorf Astoria. Wilma Rudolph, a proud, resolute, feisty woman, for all her air of gentleness, was not going to stand for that.

When the governor of Tennessee, who had been elected on a nakedly segregationist ticket, proposed a homecoming parade in her honour, she said she would take part only if it was conducted on integrated lines, with blacks and whites made equally welcome at the closing dinner. The governor, knowing when he was beaten, capitulated.

Thereafter Rudolph was in the vanguard of the campaign for civil rights in Tennessee, until the last segregationist law had been repealed. America was changing, however slowly, and after her Olympic triumph she was one of the public faces of change. FDR may have snubbed Jesse Owens. President Kennedy was not so crass, welcoming Rudolph to the White House. A great Olympian had become a national treasure.

At twenty years old, she was young enough to repeat her Rome success at Tokyo in 1964, but feeling that she had already achieved her personal ambition, she retired from athletics instead. Marriage, motherhood, a stint as a primary school teacher, a string of guest speaker engagements, her own charity, dedicated to helping underprivileged youngsters in inner-city ghettoes . . . Everything Wilma Rudolph did after Rome was of a piece with her life before Rome: a life of unceasing struggle, without vanity or histrionics, rooted in notions of service and family.

She should, by rights, have become an elder stateswoman of American sport. She should still be alive today. She would be in her seventies. But life, as Wilma Rudolph knew better than anyone, is seldom fair: if it can raise you up, it can strike you down. The Black Gazelle, the darling of millions, died of cancer in November 1994, at the age of just fifty-four. It was almost as if the natural frailty she had fought so valiantly to overcome had caught up with her. The odds, for once, were stacked so high against her that she had to admit defeat.

'When the sun is shining, I can do anything,' the athlete once said. 'No mountain is too high, no trouble too difficult.'

Her own sporting odyssey, an uphill battle that began the day she was born and ended on a podium on the other side of the world, perfectly exemplified the power of self-belief.

Eddie Paynter: 'It Were Nowt More Than a Sore Throit'

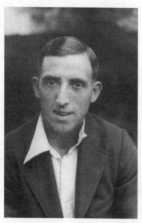

EMPICS

Lovers of sporting farce have always had a soft spot for Eddie Paynter, the pint-sized Lancastrian batsman at the centre of one of the most enchanting stories in cricketing history.

Born in unfashionable Oswaldtwistle in 1901, little Eddie was as brave as a lion, but as you read his story today, it is hard to stop yourself giggling. Half the characters seem to have walked straight out of a *Carry On* film. One of the best scenes features a man in striped pyjamas and a dressing-gown. It only needs Hattie Jacques and a bed-pan to render it complete.

As a player, Paynter was just short of the top rank. He scored a double century against Australia, which puts him in exalted company, and averaged a very impressive 59.23

in Test cricket. But in an age of batting superstars, he was
rarely in the limelight. He played twenty times for England
during the 1930s, but was in and out of the team, never
certain of his place. Compared with Hammond or Hutton,
he was a humble artisan – one who would have been long
forgotten but for the events of 13 and 14 February 1933.

The infamous Bodyline series, the most acrimonious in
cricket history, was nearing its climax. England, leading the
series 2-1, stood to regain the Ashes if they could beat
Australia in the fourth Test at the Gabba in Brisbane.

Australia won the toss and batted first, in brutal, ener-
vating heat. The England fielders started to wilt, and one of
them, it became obvious, was wilting more than the others.
Little Eddie Paynter was running a high temperature and
complaining of a sore throat. During the second day's play,
with Australia still batting, a weak and feverish Paynter was
admitted to Brisbane General Hospital and diagnosed with
acute tonsillitis. He was having difficulty breathing and
swallowing – the classic symptoms. In the pre-antibiotics
era, it was not a condition to be taken lightly.

Paynter stayed in hospital throughout the Sunday, a rest
day, when his visitors included the England captain, hard-
as-nails Douglas Jardine who, while sympathetic, impressed
on him that his services might still be needed, joking that
he would be expected to bat on crutches, if necessary.

By Monday, England had opened their innings. They
started well, posting 100 without loss in reply to 340 by
Australia, then lost wickets in a rush, subsiding to 196 for
five.

For Paynter, listening to the match on a wireless in his hospital bed, his whole life had reached its crossroads. The
doctors had told him, in no uncertain terms, that he would be
taking no further part in the Test match: acute tonsillitis was

a serious, debilitating condition, only treatable by a period of complete rest. But then the doctors *were* Australian . . .

A groggy Paynter whispered to Bill Voce, one of the England tour party, who was by his bedside, to get him a taxi. He struggled into his dressing-gown and prepared to sneak out of the hospital – only to be confronted by a very angry ward sister. When she found out that he was trying to get to the cricket ground, she 'played hell', according to Paynter, which sounds like an understatement and a half. Brisbane in the 1930s was the roughest, toughest city in Australia. One imagines the ward sister standing at six foot four, with Popeye forearms and a face like Dennis Lillee.

But the little Lancastrian was not to be cowed. When the ward sister marched off to find a doctor, he and Voce took a taxi to the Gabba, and caused a minor sensation in the England dressing-room. Jardine told Paynter to put on his pads and, when the next wicket fell, leaving England perilously placed, on 216 for six, he tottered out to the crease, clearly still weak and wearing a wide-brimmed panama as protection against the sun. In some versions of the story, which has grown with the telling, he fortified himself for the ordeal with an egg and brandy. In others, it was a few swigs of champagne.

The Australian crowd, recognising an underdog when they saw one, cheered Paynter to the echo. The Australian captain, Bill Woodfull, was sufficiently concerned by his state of health to offer him a runner – a rare gesture of sportsmanship in a series that had hitherto been contested with no quarter given by either side. Paynter, stoically, declined.

There were seventy-five minutes' playing time left in the day, and the new ball was due. The Australians had been expecting to clean up the tail and take a sizeable first-innings lead. But the Lancastrian hung in there, defending stoutly and prodding the odd single. By close of play, he was 24 not out. Still feeling terrible, he crawled back into his pyjamas and dressing-gown and was driven to the hospital, to be greeted by his nemesis, the ward sister. 'Well played,' she barked. 'Now get into bed.'

Paynter slept well, woke the next day feeling a bit better, and returned to the Gabba to resume his innings, his pockets stuffed with pills and mouth gargles. By now the Brisbane fans were cheering him as if he were an Australian. They cheered when he reached his fifty, cheered when play was suspended to allow him to gargle and take his medicine, and cheered him all the way back to the pavilion when he was finally out for 83.

He may have fallen short of a century, but he had turned the whole match on its head. Against all the odds, England had secured a first-innings lead, having looked certain to concede one. They went on to win the match by six wickets. Paynter, fittingly, hit the winning runs with a six. The Ashes had been regained.

The heroics of the man in pyjamas would have made a good sporting story at any time. In context, it was a great sporting story. In the preceding weeks and months, the Bodyline series had become the talk of the sporting world, for reasons that reflected no credit on the participants. The previous Test, in Adelaide, had marked a low point in Anglo-Australian relations, with recriminations flying. Here, suddenly, had appeared a different kind of narrative, featuring a hero whom everyone, English or Australian, could take to their hearts. People were fed up with all the name-calling: they wanted old-fashioned sporting romance.

Eddie Paynter's name was on everybody's lips, and was even mentioned in the House of Commons, to loud cheers.

When he returned to his hospital bed, he was woken up at midnight by a telephone call from his wife May, courtesy of the organisers of the Telephones and Telegraphs Exhibition in Manchester, who saw the chance to advertise their new services. Admirers in Melbourne collected £40 for him, while the many telegrams of congratulation included one from his old workmates in the Lancashire brickyard where he had been an apprentice.

When he got back to England, to his embarrassment, he received a hero's welcome. His fellow Lancastrian, Neville Cardus, doyen of cricket writers, gleefully transcribed a speech that Paynter gave at a dinner in his honour in Oxford. 'Mr Eckersley an' la-ads. Ah can't mak' any speech. Ah can only say thanks. Ah did me best at Brisbane for England an' for Lancashire. But as for talk about mi leavin' a sickbed at risk of mi dyin' – well, beggin' your pardon, Mr Eckersley, that were all rot. It were nowt more than a sore throit.'

Douglas Jardine, the captain who had visited Paynter in hospital and exhorted him to do his bit for his country, saw things rather differently. His educated mind flew back to Britain's wars in Afghanistan in the nineteenth century and 'those fellows who marched to Kandahar with fever on them' – a reference to a celebrated three-hundred-mile mountain trek led by Lord Roberts VC in August 1880. As so often in this book, sport and soldiering had become a seamless whole.

The hero of Brisbane gradually faded back into the shadows where, by temperament, he belonged. Eddie Paynter was a fine batsman, who would have walked into any England team of the last twenty years. The Second World War brought a halt to his career when he was still at the peak of his powers – he scored three centuries on the

1938–39 tour of South Africa, including a Test best 243 at Durban. But, from what we can glimpse of the man, he would have heartily detested the age of easy celebrity. The sportsmen of his generation were ordinary mortals, doing a job of work like everyone else. Paynter ended his days stacking wool in a Yorkshire mill, before dying in 1979, at the age of seventy-seven.

But he had secured his immortality. That dash to the cricket ground in pyjamas and dressing-gown perfectly embodies the heroic lunacy of sport.

Marcus Trescothick: 'How Could I Explain Something I Couldn't Understand?'

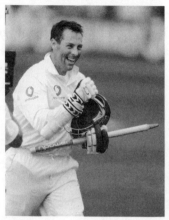

MIRRORPIX

From the dashing left-handed batsman who got off his hospital bed to win the Ashes to the dashing left-handed batsman who withdrew from an Ashes tour on grounds of stress – but had to demonstrate every bit as much courage as Eddie Paynter, maybe more.

Marcus Trescothick of Somerset was one of the most gifted players ever to open the batting for England. He scored heavily in both forms of the game and was one of the linchpins of the Ashes-winning team of 2005. But he will be remembered for non-cricketing reasons. The ruddy-faced West Country man nicknamed 'Banger' – for his uncomplicated approach to batting as much as for a weakness for sausages – was a complicated man beneath the genial surface.

Unbeknown to his England team-mates at the time, Trescothick was suffering from clinical depression, a condition that would eventually signal the end of his international career. His secret came out in a messy way. Embarrassing secrets usually do. When he had to come home early from the 2006 tour of India, the press were fobbed off with the line that he had contracted a virus, which fooled nobody. But by the time the full story came out, and Trescothick published his much-admired autobiography, *Coming Back to Me*, he was an object of sympathy throughout the cricketing world.

As an ardent Trescothick fan, I was sadder than anyone when he announced his retirement from international cricket in 2008. But I did allow myself a little smile as a hypothetical question wandered into my head. What if Trescothick had been part of the England team that toured Australia in 1932–33, the Bodyline series? How would Douglas Jardine – the captain who told Eddie Paynter he expected him to bat on crutches if necessary – have reacted if told that his opening batsman wanted to catch the next boat home because he was suffering from stress? There would have been paint peeling from the dressing-room wall.

We tend to romanticise the sportsmen of the past, with their lack of pretension and their ideals. We think of them as playing in a golden age. We forget that it was also, in some respects, a dark age, rife with bigotry and ignorance. Sport has moved on, and for the better.

Thanks, in large part, to Marcus Trescothick.

If it is hard for professional sportsmen to admit that they are gay, it can be even harder to admit that they are suffering from any form of mental illness. It goes against the grain of everything they believe in. Sports folk inhabit an earthy, unforgiving world.

When it was reported that the Rangers goalkeeper Andy Goram suffered from mild schizophrenia, the opposing fans behind the goal wasted no time in rubbing in the fact. 'There's only two Andy Gorams, two Andy Gorams . . .' Witty, arguably. Compassionate, certainly not.

When Stan Collymore checked into the Priory Clinic to be treated for depression, his Aston Villa manager, John Gregory, gave him short shrift. 'I'm very sceptical about the whole issue,' Gregory said. 'I'm of the old school, if you like. I prefer my players to roll up their sleeves and get on with life.' To the manager who had staunchly supported Paul Merson in his battle with alcoholism, depression was an illness too far – or perhaps not even an illness at all. Gregory quickly offloaded Collymore to Leicester City.

Heaven only knows what would have happened to Marcus Trescothick if he had been a footballer, not a cricketer. As it was, he got quite a rough ride in some sections of the media. In 2006, when the Somerset man first pulled out of the England team for stress-related reasons, understanding of the strains under which professional sportsmen play was still in its infancy.

In a sense, his problems should have come as no surprise. In 2001, the year after Trescothick made his international debut, David Frith published a seminal book, *Silence of the Heart*, which demonstrated that cricket had the highest suicide rate of any major sport. 'The nature of cricket is such that it tears at the nerves,' Frith wrote. 'It is the uncertainty, day in and day out, that plays a sinister beat on the cricketer's soul.' The main focus of his book was ex-players – like Yorkshire wicket-keeper David Bairstow or Jack Iverson of Australia – who took their lives after their careers were over. The idea of a current England cricketer wrestling demons that had nothing to do with his batting average or his footwork against the new ball had the horror of the unknown about it.

'Nobody knew,' says Trescothick, of the illness that for years he kept secret. 'I never told anyone about the pain I was going through because I didn't understand it myself. It made no sense to me that I felt so bad. How could I explain something I couldn't understand?'

But once he had told the world his tale, calmly and without self-pity, a little of the horror receded.

Parts of that tale were touchingly simple. On the 2005 tour of Pakistan, when Trescothick was captaining the England side, his father-in-law was taken seriously ill. His wife begged him to return home, but he put his country first. 'I was congratulated on my decision,' he remembers, 'but inside I was dying a long, slow death.' When he finally got home, his little girl, Ellie, who was a year old, did not recognise him. Small wonder that, for Trescothick, as for other cricketers, overseas tours became the most stressful times of all. And the fans probably thought he was relaxing in the sun.

But depression is not, ultimately, a simple condition. It is savagely debilitating, and can strike in random ways, at unexpected times. Trescothick could score a sparkling century, return to the pavilion with a grin on his face, then be overcome with suicidal thoughts or collapse in floods of tears. It is hard to explain that kind of emotional yo-yoing to someone who has never experienced it. You can only describe the symptoms, and trust – there can be no certainty, not in the hard-bitten world of sport – that other people will be understanding.

To their credit – and to Trescothick's relief – they were

understanding. 'I really feel for the lad,' wrote no-nonsense Yorkshireman Geoffrey Boycott in the *Daily Telegraph* when the extent of Trescothick's problems became clear. 'I know what he is going through. I opted out of playing for England for three years because it all got too much for me. When you are suffering from stress, you just want to run away. You can't face the pressure any more, and you need to escape. It is not like a broken leg or a bloody nose. There are no external symptoms and nobody can see your suffering. It is a silent illness.'

Sympathy was not confined to his fellow countrymen. After Trescothick dramatically flew home from Australia just before the start of the 2006–07 Ashes tour, the *Sydney Morning Herald* urged its readers to 'buck the tired old stereotype' of the insensitive, politically incorrect Aussie and show their sympathy for the England player. Hundreds of readers posted messages of support on the website.

In the short time since Marcus Trescothick's problems became public, there has been a sea change in attitudes. The heirs to Aston Villa manager John Gregory are still out there, but they are in a minority, emotional dinosaurs. More and more people have come to appreciate the potentially crippling stresses that lurk in the seemingly simple, wholesome life of a professional sportsman. There is a wider recognition that to admit to feeling depressed can be a sign of strength, not weakness.

We have reached a better, more compassionate place. But would we have reached it, even now, if one brave cricketer had not shown the way?

Trescothick's spanking cover drives were one of the most glorious sights in cricket. But his main legacy to sport is what he achieved off the field.

Randy Romero:
A Flipping Marvel

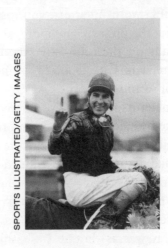

Somewhere in the United States, under lock and key in a doctor's surgery, lies a medical file on jockey Randy Romero. It must be at least six inches thick by now, and getting thicker every year.

'He's the bionic man of racing,' his wife Cricket once told an interviewer. 'You tell me a bone and Randy has broken it.'

Between 1975 and 1994, the jockey known as the 'Ragin' Cajun' rode more than four thousand winners and earned over $70 million dollars. He was one of the best in the business, although his career was dogged by injury after injury, and he required surgery on more than twenty separate occasions. Fans said the Ragin' Cajun was jinxed – while warming to a gutsy competitor who never seemed to know when he was beaten.

In 1983 the jockey suffered 65 per cent burns in a freak accident in a sauna during a race meeting in Arkansas. He had rubbed himself down with alcohol, then accidentally broken a light bulb, causing his whole body to go up in flames: it took him more than six months to recuperate. His other injuries were less dramatic, but no less harrowing.

Of his many falls on the race-track, the most famous occurred in the Breeders' Cup Distaff race in 1990, when his mount, Go for Wand, fell fifty yards from the finish. The horse had broken its foreleg and had to be put down. Romero was treated in hospital for bruised ribs and was back in the saddle after four races. Several days later X-rays revealed that he had actually broken eight of his ribs and cracked a shoulder.

In Florida the following year, the jockey had another fall, suffering concussion, a broken left elbow and a fractured collarbone. It was as though his body were being continually dismantled and reassembled, like something in Dr Frankenstein's laboratory. He had screws in his shoulders and ankles, and a steel plate on the left side of his face. His spleen had been removed. He had broken his femur. All because he had been horse-mad since he was a kid growing up in Louisiana.

'Randy is basically immune to pain,' his wife told reporters in 1991. 'He's an optimist. He says pain goes with the territory. He knows the consequences. I worry about him, but he loves riding, and I could never ask him to give it up.'

A doctor thumbing through his file at that time would have had no problem making a diagnosis. Professional jockey, vulnerable to the occupational hazards of his profession, viz. falling off horses. Fragile of build, therefore multiple fractures inevitable, but possesses exceptional resilience and determination. Wants to get back in the saddle at the earliest opportunity. Slightly mad, like most sportsmen, but brave as a lion and a model professional.

Only a very alert doctor would have spotted Randy Romero's real problem, which came to light after he had retired.

Go back to that sauna accident in Arkansas in 1983. The incident with the broken light bulb is so exotic that it distracts attention from the question that the medically curious might otherwise ask themselves. What kind of person takes a sauna in Arkansas, a Southern state where the humidity is so high that even walking down the street feels like a visit to a Turkish bath?

Answer: a professional jockey obsessed to the point of clinical disorder with keeping his weight down.

Never mind the broken bones. Randy Romero was seriously ill.

Every sport has its grubby secrets, and in horse racing, where race-fixing scandals tend to hog the limelight, one of the grubbiest secrets of all has gone largely unreported. Randy Romero's full medical story, and its implications for his sport, came out only when he took part in a TV documentary in 2004.

The jockey had announced his retirement in 1994, at the comparatively early age of thirty-seven, citing long-term liver and kidney damage. In 2002, his kidneys started to fail, and he was told that he had Hepatitis C, which raised further complications, as it ruled out a liver or kidney transplant. His liver subsequently stabilised, and he was put on a course of kidney dialysis, but the prognosis was grim. What the world did not know, until the documentary, was that Romero, like many of his fellow jockeys, had suffered from acute bulimia throughout his career, vomiting five or six times a day. He had been abusing his body for years, desperate to keep his weight down to the level demanded under American racing rules – around 113 pounds, even lower than weight limits in the UK.

'The bulimia is as bad as being a cocaine addict,' Romero calmly confessed, on prime time television. 'It works on your nervous system. It works on your mind. I put 150 per cent into riding, but it got me into the position I am in now.'

Jockey, screened on HBO, lifted the lid on an entire subculture in the weighing-room: as disturbing as, though far less familiar than, the similar subculture in the world of catwalk models. The practice of 'flipping' – jockey-speak for vomiting – is apparently so ubiquitous in America that, at many race-tracks, 'heaving bowls' are located in the changing rooms for general use. Win a race, eat, chuck up. There can hardly be a group of sportsmen anywhere in the world who lead such an abnormal existence.

'I had no control,' says Romero, describing some of the classic symptoms of an eating disorder. 'I was hungry all the time.' Most weeks, he would be lucky if he kept down two meals all week. He also went through periods of alcohol abuse. 'I'm not proud of what I did,' he admitted. 'I should have been a lot smarter.' But there were few in the money-obsessed world of horse racing available to offer him advice and support when he most needed it.

The health risks for weight-obsessed jockeys are obvious, medically, and have been known about in general terms for some time. A 1995 study by the Chicago Rehabilitation Unit found that 35 per cent of jockeys used diuretics;

30 per cent vomited regularly; 67 per cent tried to sweat off weight in saunas; and 14 per cent resorted to laxatives. But until the 2004 documentary, in which Romero and another Louisiana jockey, Shane Sellers, came clean, there had been a conspiracy of silence, broken only by isolated horror stories.

In 1991 the Australian Supreme Court had ruled that a jockey who suffered a heart attack in a sauna was entitled to substantial damages. In 2000 an American jockey had died of heart arrhythmia after his potassium levels plummeted as a result of dieting. Yet it needed a big-name jockey like Romero, someone who could talk frankly about his own experiences, to raise the profile of the issue. His candid confessions may have shocked a few people, but they made it a good deal harder to brush the whole subject under the carpet.

In an interview in 2008, by which time his health was steadily deteriorating, Romero vowed to devote the remainder of his life to leading calls for curbs on weight limits for jockeys.

'Look at the position I am in,' he told the interviewer. 'I could die and the weight system would have a lot to do with it. I'd hate to see anyone go through what I'm going through.'

The present limits date back to the mid-nineteenth century, when the average human being was significantly lighter. So there is a prima facie case for an increase of five pounds or so. But heavier jockeys would significantly increase the risk of injuries to horses – which is why some top trainers continue to oppose them.

Whatever the future holds, the Ragin' Cajun has rewritten the terms of the debate with his courage and honesty. Fans loved him because he was a daredevil jockey: falling off his horse and remounting, again and again, as soon as the doctors gave him the all-clear. Now, in challenging doctors to ask different questions of the jockeys in their care, rather than going into denial, he has paved the way for a more compassionate attitude to a deep-seated problem.

Derek Redmond: 'I Felt a Hand on My Shoulder'

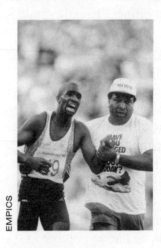

EMPICS

Courage or idiocy? Again and again in this book, the two have become indistinguishable. In the heat of the moment, sportsmen and women have taken leave of their senses, recklessly subjecting their bodies to punishment in a way that borders on the ridiculous. When one looks for their counterparts on the battlefield, it is not the heroes of the D-Day landings that come to mind, risking all in a noble cause, but the heroes of the Charge of the Light Brigade, risking all in an idiotic cause. 'Someone had blundered.'

The idiocy doesn't diminish the courage. If anything, it magnifies it. A large part of sport's charm is its ability simultaneously to stir contrasting emotions. It can make you leap to your feet clapping and cheering and, in the same instant, make you laugh. Laugh that so much passion has been expended in such a trivial cause. Laugh at the confidence trick – the illusion that the result matters – that has fooled the watching spectators. Sport is not grand opera, however much it puffs and pants. It is theatre of the absurd.

No actor in that theatre has expressed its illogical beauty better than British runner Derek Redmond, the clown-hero of the Barcelona Olympics in 1992. The footage of his doomed bid to reach the 400m final has become more celebrated than many famous sporting victories. When the organisers of the Beijing Olympics were looking for exemplars of sporting courage to use in promotional videos, Redmond was one of the first athletes to feature.

He was an outstanding runner. In 1985, and again in 1987, he broke the British 400m record. At the 1991 World Championships he was part of the British 4 × 400m relay team that caused a major upset by beating the Americans. His career was dogged by setbacks. At the 1988 Olympics in Seoul, he had to pull out of the opening round of the 400m, just before the start, because of an injury to his Achilles tendon. A long series of operations followed. But Redmond was not a quitter: he was a survivor. He resumed training, started to win again, pushed his body to its limits. When he lined up in the 400m semi-final in Barcelona, having already won his quarter-final, he seemed certain to qualify for the final.

The torn hamstring that ended his race was just one of those things. It was dramatic in its sheer suddenness, an audible snap that brought Redmond to a juddering halt. 'I thought I had been shot,' he later recalled. But it was not unprecedented, nor medically remarkable. Just a run-of-the-mill sporting injury, you would have said, if it had not been for what happened next – Redmond deciding that, torn hamstring or not, he was going to finish the race.

As he hobbled down the home straight, the spectators were so bemused that they were not sure how to react. There was embarrassment in the air, a sense that the British runner had lost the plot and was about to make a complete fool of himself. Ahead of Redmond, the race had already finished. What was the point of carrying on running? This was not courage. It was rank stupidity. Or headless-chicken syndrome, the body continuing to do its own thing, severed from the brain.

In an instant, the stupid was elevated to the sublime.

A man in shorts and a T-shirt rushed out of the crowd. To the spectators in the stadium, he was a stranger, his identity a riddle, his motives obscure. But the TV viewers back in England – who included myself, watching the race from my sofa – were more fortunate. The commentator recognised the man immediately. He was no stranger, but an actor whose sudden appearance made perfect sense. He was Redmond's father Jim, the man who had supported him throughout his career.

'Everything I had worked for was finished,' remembers Derek Redmond. 'I hated everybody. I hated the world. I hated hamstrings. I felt so bitter I was injured again. I told myself I had to finish. I kept hopping round. Then I felt a hand on my shoulder. It was my old man.'

Jim Redmond, for his part, could have remonstrated with his son, tried to dissuade him from finishing the race. That is what many parents would have done, faced with a child doing something toe-curlingly embarrassing. Jim Redmond, magnificently, did not try to stop his son making a fool of himself. He helped him make a fool of himself. He made himself an accomplice to his stupidity.

Brushing aside a marshal who tried to stop him, he put his arm around his son's shoulder, and the two men staggered towards the line together, like a couple of drunks, cheered on by the Barcelona crowd, who were by now totally captivated. Tears were streaming down Derek Redmond's face, but the mood in the stadium was upbeat: something had been retrieved from the wreckage. Out of bitter disappointment, one of the noblest chapters in the history of sport had been written.

In the folklore of athletics, Derek Redmond will be forever associated with the runner who finishes, come what may. Sports fans, as a general rule, do not like quitters. When Paula Radcliffe broke down and failed to finish the marathon at the 2004 Olympics in Athens, she was roundly criticised. In athletics, the runners finishing fourth and fifth, or even twenty-fourth or twenty-fifth, give context and meaning to the achievements of the runners on the podium.

Derek Redmond limping towards the finishing-line in Barcelona has become an emblem of the sportsman for whom it is not the winning, but the taking part, that counts. Since retiring from athletics, he has been in demand as a motivational speaker, and no wonder.

Yet for raw courage, inspirational steadfastness, his father shares the podium with him. What a beautiful parable of the parental journey. You raise your child, nurture him, encourage him, help him try to achieve his dreams. But when he is a grown man and making a fool of himself, you don't turn your back on him. You are there for him, as you have been since he drew his first breath.

Parents the world over grit their teeth and stand by their children when they make fools of themselves. But not many of them have had to do it on such a public stage as Jim Redmond. Under a Barcelona sun, an English father set an example to fathers everywhere.

Team Hoyt: The Indomitables

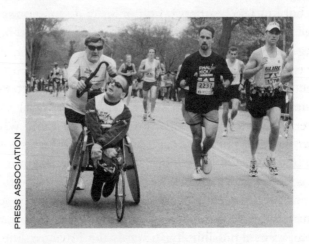

PRESS ASSOCIATION

Jim Redmond helping his son across the finishing-line in Barcelona was sport in miniature, a hastily improvised drama that was over almost before the spectators had worked out who the characters were. Thanks to television, footage of the race has now been watched by millions, and achieved iconic status. But the footage is too fleeting to linger, the way other sporting dramas linger.

For an undeniable epic of sporting courage, in which a father and son again take centre stage, it is necessary to cross the Atlantic and contemplate the unparalleled thirty-year odyssey of Dick and Rick Hoyt – or, as they are now universally known, Team Hoyt. Their story is better known in the States than in this country, and has been stirringly told in *It's Only a Mountain* by Sam Nall. But their

nationality is an irrelevance. Sporting heroism of this mag-
nitude knows no boundaries.

Dick Hoyt, a resident of Massachusetts, is a retired
Lieutenant Colonel in the Air National Guard. His son
Rick, born in 1962, suffers from cerebral palsy, a condition
that occurs when the flow of oxygen to the brain is blocked
during birth. In Rick's case, his umbilical cord became
badly twisted around his neck, condemning him, according
to doctors, to live in a permanent vegetative state. They
recommended placing him in an institution, but Rick's
mother, Judy Hoyt, was having none of it. 'There is no
way we will ever put our son away,' she said. 'We love him.
He is ours. We will work with him and bring him to the
place where he can achieve his greatest potential.'

For the next fifteen years, step by patient step, the Hoyts
did just that, giving their son a better quality of life than
had ever seemed possible. They played with him, took him
swimming, taught him the alphabet by posting signs on
every object in the house. When schools refused to take
him, on the grounds that he was unable to communicate,
they worked with the engineering department of a university to devise a computer that would enable Rick to
articulate the thoughts he could not speak. A cursor was
attached to his head – one of the few parts of his body he
could move freely – which allowed him to activate a special
touch pad. Soon fully formed sentences were starting to
appear, and he was admitted to school.

As the Hoyts had long suspected, their son proved to be
academically bright, and would later graduate from university with a degree in special education. 'My hope,' he
said, 'is that by seeing what I can do, and listening to my
achievements, all people, and especially young people, will
see that I am just like them.' Yet it was not Rick Hoyt's

academic progress that captured the public imagination, but his engagement with sport.

When he first went to school, he would be wheeled to the library instead of attending PE classes. But an enterprising gym teacher called Dr Steve Sartori had other ideas. He encouraged Rick to take part in physical activities with other students, then invited him to attend a basketball game, where Rick spotted a sign advertising a five-mile charity fun-run. 'Dad, I want to do that,' Rick tapped out, in a message to his father. An astonished Dick Hoyt did his best to grant his son's wish, pushing him the length of the course in a wheelchair. As he was not particularly fit, nobody expected Team Hoyt to get past the first corner, let alone finish the race.

But they did finish – and have gone on finishing for the last thirty years, participating in over a thousand events, including more than fifty marathons.

Between them, they have mastered a whole range of disciplines, including the triathlon, where Dick pulls his son in a special boat, carries him in a special seat on a bicycle, then pushes him in a specially designed wheelchair. His never-say-die determination has won him admirers all over the world. Even after he suffered a heart attack in 2003, he did not throw in the towel. The next year, Team Hoyt was back where it had left off, competing in the Boston Marathon.

Why do they do it? In a nutshell, because the words Rick Hoyt tapped out to his father after that first race, in the spring of 1977, were a call to arms: 'Dad, when I'm running, it feels like I'm not handicapped.' What father could fail to respond to such a cue? 'Making Rick happy,' in the words of Dick Hoyt, 'was the greatest feeling in the world.'

The heroics of Team Hoyt could be the ultimate sporting

feel-good story, a triumph of the human spirit in the teeth of adversity. But sporting parables are seldom that simple. Dick and Rick Hoyt were destined to pay a heavy price for their single-mindedness.

In 1992, in their most ambitious venture yet, they participated in a 45-day, 3753-mile, bike-and-run trek across the United States. But the mammoth, eye-catching journey was all too much for Judy Hoyt, Rick's mother, who felt alienated and frustrated, believing that her indefatigable husband was pushing her son too far. Their marriage ended shortly afterwards.

Did she have a point? Was there something unhealthy in this restless striving towards new goals? It would be impertinent to speculate. Sport has always driven people to their physical limits, and sometimes beyond them. That is the nature of the beast. If it were only practised by people who were of sound mind, it would be very dull for the spectators. We need the passions, the excesses, the madness.

Rick Hoyt, determined not to let his life be blighted by cerebral palsy, stands in the same tradition. When he was still at school, he wrote an essay in which he articulated his needs and frustrations with touching clarity: 'I understand everything that is said to me. Being a non-vocal person does not make one less of a human being. I have the same feelings as everyone else. I feel sadness, joy, hunger, love, compassion, pain . . .'

Sport, ultimately, gave him the stage to reveal the range and depth of those feelings. We should not exaggerate the role it plays in life, but then neither should we be coy in affirming that. A seventy-year-old man pushing his son in a wheelchair, sweat pouring down both their faces, is not an aberration: it is an inspiration.

Peter Norman: The Lone Soldier

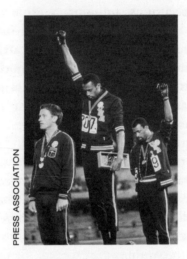

PRESS ASSOCIATION

When Australian sprinter Peter Norman finished second in the 200m at the Mexico Olympics, he went through the range of emotions familiar to every sportsman who has ever been a runner-up. So near and yet so far . . .

It would not be his national anthem played at the medals ceremony. The ultimate glory had eluded him. But why wallow in disappointment? Why not take pride in what he had achieved? There was no disgrace in silver. Nobody back in Australia had expected him to win any kind of medal. His time was a personal best and a national record, which still stands. Not bad for a former apprentice butcher from Melbourne.

Norman had no way of knowing that, in the next two hours, his life would be turned upside down.

That he would be faced with a stark choice, and make the right choice, but be reviled for the choice he made.

That he would go to his grave, nearly forty years later, without getting a fraction of the credit his courage deserved.

Who would be a successful sportsman?

The story of Peter Norman, the third man on the podium at Mexico City in 1968, would have been largely forgotten, to all our shames, if it had not been turned into a movie by his nephew, Matt Norman. *Salute* was released in 2008 and, although not a big hit at the box office, reminded the world of a remarkable and brave individual.

To the millions watching the 1968 Olympics on television, Norman was so comprehensively upstaged by the two men who shared the podium with him that nobody looked at him twice. All eyes were riveted on Tommie Smith and John Carlos, whose clenched-fist Black Power salutes reverberated around the world.

People missed one small but significant detail: the badge of the Olympic Project for Human Rights (OPHR), a States-wide civil rights protest movement, which Norman was wearing as a gesture of solidarity with his fellow athletes.

How did a young man from Melbourne get so entangled in American politics? Everything happened in a chaotic whirl, in the short time between the race and the medals ceremony. Smith and Carlos confided to Norman that they were planning to make a protest on the podium, and the Australian was, in part, responsible for the choreography. The Americans originally both planned to raise two gloved fists while the Stars and Stripes was played. Unfortunately, John Carlos had left his gloves in the Olympic Village. 'Why not wear one glove each?' suggested Norman. Hence the now iconic, oddly lopsided, image of Smith raising his right fist and Carlos his left.

And the Australian's involvement did not end there. As the three athletes made their way through the tunnel to the medal ceremony, a well-wisher in the stands offered Norman an OPHR badge, which he immediately, and without hesitation, pinned to his tracksuit. The die was cast. The podium beckoned.

'I'm a firm believer,' Norman said, years later, 'that in a victory ceremony for the Olympics, there's three guys that stand up there, each one's been given a square metre of God's earth to stand on, and what any one of the three chooses to do with his little square metre at that stage is entirely up to him.'

As far as the athlete was concerned, he was just doing the instinctive, decent thing. He was a Christian. His family had been involved with the Salvation Army for generations. 'I believe in civil rights,' he would tell reporters afterwards. 'Every man is born equal and should be treated that way.' But associating himself with such a controversial gesture, guaranteed to outrage the Olympic authorities, was asking for trouble.

The punishments meted out to Smith and Carlos were swift and savage. Both men were sent home from Mexico in disgrace. Their athletic careers were as good as over. In time, they would become folk heroes, but not before they had paid a high price in their personal lives, receiving a torrent of death threats and hate mail. The strain on John Carlos and his family became intolerable, and his wife eventually committed suicide in 1977. Tommie Smith was briefly reduced to washing cars for a living. His mother died of a heart attack after being sent manure and dead rats in the post by white farmers.

For Peter Norman, retribution for his part in the protest followed more slowly. The Australia of his day was, if anything, even less sympathetic to the cause of racial integration and tolerance than the United States. Only in 1962 were Aborigines given voting rights in federal elections; only in 1967 were they included in the national census. In showing solidarity with Tommie Smith and John Carlos, Norman could hardly have chosen associates less likely to endear him to his fellow countrymen.

He escaped with a slap on the wrist at Mexico City, but as far as the Australian Olympic Committee was concerned, had become *persona non grata*, and would remain so until his death. He would normally have been an automatic selection for the 1972 Olympics in Munich, having run well within the qualifying time, but was left at home: the powers-that-be were afraid of a repetition of the Mexico protest.

For a time, Norman worked as a teacher and sports coach, as well as playing football for West Brunswick, but considering that he was an Olympic medallist, was fast slipping into sporting oblivion. In 1985 he contracted gangrene in his Achilles tendon and nearly had to have his leg amputated; after that, he fell into a profound depression, became addicted to painkillers, and had to battle alcoholism, committing a string of drink-driving offences.

By the time of the 2000 Olympics in Sydney, he was a virtual pariah. Other former Australian Olympians were included in the various special events and ceremonies, but Norman, pointedly, was ignored. Is there anything that scares sports administrators as much as a maverick, a nonconformist? A new, racially tolerant Australia was about to be unveiled to the world, epitomised by Cathy Freeman carrying the Olympic flame; but nobody seemed able to make the connection with that symbolic, eye-catching statement and the quiet rebel of Mexico City.

Norman's rehabilitation owed more to American sense of fair play than to Australian public opinion. When the American delegation to Sydney heard that Norman had not received an invitation to the Games, they insisted that he come as their guest. The reverence with which he was now viewed in the States was encapsulated by the great Michael Johnson, who, on being introduced to the Australian, said simply: 'You are my hero.'

In 2005, when a twenty-foot bronze statue of the famous clenched-fist salute was unveiled at San Jose State University, which Carlos and Smith had attended, Peter Norman was one of the guests of honour. 'It's an honour to call these men my friends,' he said, draping his arms around their shoulders.

A year later, he was dead, of a heart attack, and the debt of friendship had to be paid for the last time. Carlos and Smith both flew to Melbourne and were pallbearers at his funeral at Williamstown Town Hall, where Carlos gave a eulogy of heartfelt simplicity:

> As we stand here thinking about Peter Norman, think about the greatness of the man who said: 'I stand with you. I don't stand before you, I don't stand behind you, but I stand with you.'
>
> He was a lone soldier in Australia. Many people in Australia didn't particularly understand. Why would that young white fella go over and stand with those black individuals? Peter was Australian and he was proud to be Australian. He was proud to run and represent Australia. But even greater than that, he said: 'I'm proud to represent the human race.' I stand in awe of him.

Even in 2011, that sense of awe is not widely shared in Australia, where Peter Norman is less celebrated than a thousand far less worthy sportsmen. But there, in miniature, is the pathos that so often accompanies courage.

You do the right thing or what, in the heat of the moment, seems to be the right thing. You don't get any medals for doing it. You just have to trust your heart, and hope for a fair hearing afterwards. To be courageous, in some sporting contexts, can make you a hero overnight. More often, it simply isolates you, condemns you to an uncertain future. Courage can be the loneliest of all the virtues.

Of the sportsmen and women featured in this book, probably only a minority would classify as red-blooded sporting heroes, the kind that used to sell comic books. Bert Trautmann fitted the mould. So, in their different ways, did Eric Liddell, Eddie Paynter, Jackie Robinson, Lis Hartel, Walter Hagen and, in more recent times, Niki Lauda, Dean Jones, Grant Hackett and Ellie Simmonds. But most of the others trod a far more uncertain path, dividing opinion or, in some cases, scandalising it. They put their careers on the line when they did not need to. They got hate mail amid the fan letters.

They thought the sporting life would be one grand sweet song. When they became professional sportsmen, they had to pinch themselves that they were being paid for something they would have done for love. They glimpsed the pitfalls of sporting celebrity only gradually. People demanded that they behave like role models, but nobody told them what a role model was, or how notions of what was right and wrong, acceptable and unacceptable, would change from day to day, season to season. They had to grope their way through the moral maze as best they could.

Peter Norman's journey through that maze took him far from his comfort zone as an athlete. But, as with the other men and women remembered here, when his courage was put to the test, he did not falter.